God is in Your Full-Length Mirror

Five biblical steps to lifetime weight loss

by Heidi Fingar, M.P.H.

www.YourFullLengthMirror.com

God is in Your Full-Length Mirror

Five biblical steps to lifetime weight loss

by Heidi Fingar, M.P.H.

PUBLISHED BY

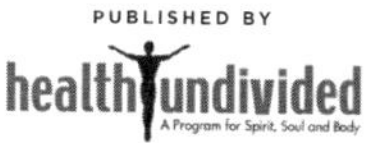

God is in Your Full-Length Mirror

Published by Health Undivided, Hilton Head Island, SC 29928

ISBN 978-0-6153253-7-8

Library of Congress Control Number: 2009910866

Editors:
Kathleen Fuller
Gerhard Gartner

Design and manufacturing:

Lydia Inglett Design, Publishing & Print Management

Printed in China

www.YourFullLengthMirror.com

Heartfelt thanks to Jeanine Siebold, Jim Moore, Kathleen Fuller, Pastor Gilbert Posey and my dad, Gerhard Gartner, for their many hours of editing and theological counsel. Special thanks to the countless family, friends and clients that gave me the courage to finish this book... and to my husband, Walt, for the sacrifices he has made to help me realize my dreams - I love you Honig.

Greatest thanks to my Lord, Savior and best friend, Jesus Christ, for He loved me first and gave me this path of healing.

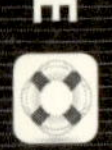

Contents

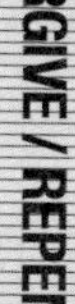

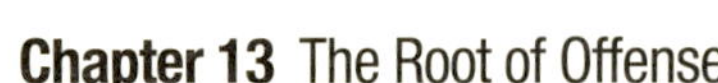

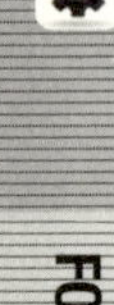

RELEASE
EXAMINE
EXPRESS
RECOGNIZE

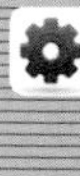

FORGIVE / REPENT

Introduction

Staring back at me from pictures in an old photo album is a face I recognize. I feel sadness as I recount the details of her life. She appears to be of average weight yet she wears clothes that hide her figure – large, baggy sweaters and t-shirts; shorts reaching to the middle of her knees, hiding her shapely form. Even in a picture at her 23rd birthday celebration, she covers her body in a black skirt, black tights and an oversized sweater. She is fashionable in her attire but I know that pastels and prints, and a form-fitted top would be more than appropriate for this special occasion. In fact, I know that she loves other colors but she doesn't dare to wear anything but black (especially on her bottom half).

I look at her closely and her eyes remind me of an agonizing battle. To her friends and family she seems to be happy but she is distracted. Her enemy, present at every party and social function, is demanding far more attention than any one person or conversation. She is at war. This battle takes her to the trenches of her soul, demanding her focus and energy.

Every day this girl fights with food. The storm rages from the moment she rises to the moment she goes to bed. In the morning, she skips breakfast and runs several miles before anyone else is out of bed or she eats a piece of dry toast and then teaches a couple hours of aerobics classes. Each night she binges on whatever food is available in her home. Since she keeps "bad food" out of the cupboards, she has to concoct treats that satisfy her cravings – oatmeal mixed with butter and chocolate baking squares, heated in the microwave, or popcorn coated with butter spray and hot cocoa powder. On the nights she hosts the youth group at her house, she finishes off the remaining pizza, pulling leftover crusts from the garbage and leftover ice cream from the freezer. Then there are the nights she simply steals things from her roommate's side of the kitchen – leftover Chinese, chips and salsa, saltines and cheese – whatever is available.

Sometimes the food tastes good, but most of the time, she doesn't notice the taste. If it fills her, she's satisfied. Even in sleep, she's tormented with nightmares of binge eating and gaining weight, only to wake up and find she didn't really eat the gobs of food in her dreams. Then she is up and running, literally, as she works through her day again, burning calories and guilt, caused by the nightly binge. The cycle of daily starving and night-time feeding continues for years and there is no relief in sight.

I'm the woman in the photo album. For over twenty years, I personally fought with overeating. In my quest for answers addressing binge eating, I scoured the conventional methods offered for change and came up wanting. Attempting to find the solution in countless weight loss programs, I only found myself losing weight then gaining it back again. I ate pre-ordered meals in plastic packaging, cut out the fat, eliminated the carbs and fasted in long intervals. None of these methods offered me the answers I craved.

So I surrounded myself with other health enthusiasts. I worked in fitness centers and gyms for twelve years in management, as an exercise class instructor, and as a personal trainer. I gained certifications in every form of exercise that came along, studying books on physiology, nutrition and exercise. I coached, goaded and encouraged thousands of weight loss seekers in swimming pools, toning classes, kickboxing, and step aerobics. I pounded the pavement in six-mile runs, lifted weights five to six days a week, and competed in triathlons and half marathons.

In all of those years, I tried answering the repetitive questions my clients would pose regarding weight loss, diet and exercise. I gave the same answers others had given me. Then I would witness clients of mine lose weight, and, like me, gain it back again. I started to become discouraged in my work, knowing that I was not able to help others find permanent change in lifestyle and health. The deeper discouragement was that I too was looking vainly for the same answers.

In the last four years of this time span, while studying for my master's degree in Public Health, I applied behavior change theories to my work, consulting with overweight people one on one. I started a weight management group that met each week and we experienced some success together. We applied the "textbook" answers to our struggles with food. We found some help in this application, but still, the life changing answers lay undiscovered.

Throughout these years of searching, I also went before God repeatedly, seeking answers from Him, asking Him to help me in my struggle with food and rescue me from this fight. I see now that during that time, I wasn't truly open to receiving the answers He had for me. I wasn't ready to face the reality of my overeating and to see it from His perspective.

In 2001, I began to enter into a season of depression and I became desperate for help. At that point, God responded to my lifetime prayer and began to unveil His steps of freedom from bondage to food. Through a miraculous series of events and levels of revelation, in a way only God could author, He broke the weight loss/weight gain cycle over my life. When I started applying God's truth to my overeating, my life drastically changed. I began to find a peace with food I had never before experienced. My intimacy with God and others increased and I found new joy.

The five steps He gave me are simple and they stand upon Bible-based principles that specifically relate to a compulsive relationship with food. Yet you can apply these same steps to any negative behavior with ensuing success. I have shared these five steps with others and together, we have witnessed deep, lasting change. These successes prove the effectiveness of these timeless, biblical truths applied practically to overeating. In this book, I outline these steps in hopes that the healing will continue for anyone that is open to receiving them.

If you relate in any way to this sort of struggle, I invite you to read through my process of healing. Along the way, I will share the healing God has given me and testimonies from others that too have experienced lasting change.

I look at pictures today of the pretty woman that once wore over-sized sweaters and black pants and she is now wearing white shorts and pink, sleeveless tops. Her eyes are shining, her face is peaceful. Her days are hopeful and her nights are without bingeing. Food nightmares are nonexistent and dreams of success are becoming reality. She has been healed of the binge/diet cycle and she has a story to tell. She wants to share with you God's plan for healing.

If you struggle with the role food has held in your life, this may be too hard to believe. You can trust me that it's true. But if you can't trust me directly, trust God in me. He loves you. He is in your full-length mirror.

Chapter 1

The Definition of Normal Eating

According to the latest statistics, over half of all adult Americans are overweight and a third are obese. 20 to 50 percent of these same people suffer from binge eating.[1,2] There are a vast number of solutions that address binge eating, yet the number of people struggling with this disorder continues to increase each year. The conventional diets, pills and programs are not proving effective in helping us achieve deep and lasting results.

However, in order to understand abnormal behavior, we must first define normal behavior. God created us with a necessity to eat and drink while we live on this earth. The Bible also reveals that He has blessed us by giving us appropriate food and drink for our benefit in two distinct, but closely connected ways. One use is physical health and the other is celebration.

PHYSICAL HEALTH

By consuming nutritious food and drink, we sustain physical health and experience increases in energy and strength. In the book of Genesis, we read that God gave humankind every seed-bearing plant on the face of the earth for food. After the flood of Noah, God also gave humankind all wild animals, birds and fish to eat as well. The purpose for food – and one of God's original purposes – is to bring health and sustenance to the human body.

CELEBRATION

Secondly, since God made humans for fellowship, He has provided food and drink to foster this interaction through celebration. Not only is food nutritious for our physical bodies but it can also be edifying to our souls. God wants us to celebrate life and the fruit of our labors, savoring the taste of that fruit and the satisfaction that accompanies it.

In the book of Ecclesiastes, King Solomon shares his search for meaning and satisfaction during the days God granted him to live on earth. In his quest, he makes a concerted effort to experience passion, work and wisdom at extreme levels in order to gain meaning in his life. But in all three cases he only finds bitter, unsatisfying ends. After each of these futile attempts, he repeats four times a revelation he learns that includes the use of food and drink:

"So I concluded that there is nothing better for people than to be happy and to enjoy themselves as long as they can. And people should eat and drink and enjoy the fruits of their labor, for these are gifts from God." (NLT)[3]

I agree. The enjoyment of eating and drinking is a gift from God. It adds pleasure and contentment to our lives and often works in tandem with celebration to promote fellowship and to build relationships. Feasting is central to every wedding, birthday party, national holiday, religious celebration and family reunion, and remains a critical part.

After looking at the effect of celebration and energy offered by food, we can see that God gave food as a gift to humankind to add health to our spirits, souls and bodies.

THE DEFINITION OF BINGE EATING

Now that we've defined the normal use of food as God intended, we can look at abnormal uses of food. The American Psychiatric Association (APA) considers binge eating as a psychiatric illness with specific criteria including the following:

1. Consuming extremely large amounts of food, totaling several thousand calories, in a short period of time
2. Consuming food rapidly
3. Recurring episodes of binge eating – at least twice a week over six months
4. Bingeing alone
5. Feeling a lack of control or inability to stop during a binge
6. Post-binge feelings of self-hatred, guilt, depression or disgust
7. No purging, fasting, excessive exercise or other compensation for calories ingested.[4]

The APA defines a similar eating disorder, *Bulimia Nervosa*, as follows:

A. Recurrent episodes of binge eating. An episode of binge eating is characterized by both of the following:

1. eating, in a discrete period of time (e.g., within any 2-hour period), an amount of food that is definitely larger than most people would eat during a similar period of time and under similar circumstances,
2. a sense of lack of control over eating during the episode (e.g., a feeling that one cannot stop eating or control what or how much one is eating)

B. Recurrent inappropriate compensatory behavior in order to prevent weight gain, such as self-induced vomiting; misuse of laxatives, diruetics, enemas, or other medications; fasting; or excessive exercise.

C. The binge eating and inappropriate compensatory behavior both occur, on average, at least twice a week for 3 months.

D. Self-evaluation is unduly influenced by body shape and weight.[5]

The criteria goes on to explain that there are two types, purging and non-purging. People that suffer from the non-purging type use fasting or excessive exercise. This is the way I compensated for excessive calories. I believe that dieting is one other form of compensation that should be considered for people with non-purging eating disorders. Those with Binge Eating Disorder (B.E.D.), similar to those with anorexia nervosa and bulimia, are obsessed with food and use it as a drug to offer temporary solutions for emotional issues. Yet unlike bulimia and anorexia, people with B.E.D. are usually overweight or obese because they don't compensate for their bingeing with laxatives, purging, over-exercising or periods of starvation. B.E.D is a serious disorder that steals health from individuals, impacting them at physical, emotional, economic and social levels.

Though the criteria defined by the APA for these two eating disorders may seem extreme, most of us act out the above listed behaviors at some level. Perhaps you are not clinically classified with an eating disorder, but even at a sub-clinical level, eating disorders can wreak havoc in your life. Simply being preoccupied with thoughts of what your next meal will consist of can lead to great inner frustration.

I consider any eating done in an effort to comfort oneself as bingeing.

Since this definition for "bingeing" is the same when describing overeating or emotional eating, I use these three terms interchangeably. Though this definition is far more encompassing than most, it is worth our attention because the problems of sub-clinical eating disorders are rarely addressed with seriousness.

Before God started showing me His plan for eating, I suffered from the non-purging type of bulimia. I binged at night and then ate meager meals in the daytime while exercising over an hour almost every day, some days, working out two hours and more. I was known as a very tough exercise instructor and I took great pride in working my participants to exhaustion. If I overate especially bad the day before a class, my poor students would suffer along with me as I sweated off the calories and the guilt for my prior night's behavior.

The consequences of these actions were always negative. There was ensuing guilt, a lowered self-esteem, a decrease in energy, and eventually, in my future, there would be an increase in risk factors for disease. I also suffered from injury caused by overuse. In fact, I can no longer run or perform high impact exercise due to a back injury I have gained by pounding on my joints every day.

I wasn't eating to give my body health and energy and I wasn't eating in celebration for the work I did. I ate in an effort to comfort myself. The emotions I stuffed down with food ranged from sadness to anger and from disappointment to disbelief. Then I would compensate for these excess calories with exercise and dieting.

These methods I used to make up for my overeating looked normal because dieting and exercise are greatly encouraged by our society. Yet, I was not normal. I was killing myself. I was just doing it at a slower speed and at a deep, unobserved level. Others may have seen that I was unhappy with myself but they could not put a finger on the source of my unhappiness.

I always thought that friends and family were not affected by my extreme behavior, but at an indirect level, everyone I knew suffered. This is because overeating does not stand alone. There are results to this type of negative behavior that cannot be ignored. Let's look at some of them and the moral implications attached to emotional eating in the next chapter.

---

[1] B. Bruce and D. Wilfley. Binge eating among overweight population: A serious and prevalent problem *Journal of the American Dietetic Association* 96 (1996): 58-61.

[2] R.L. Spitzer, M. Devlin, B.T. Walsch, D. Hasin, R. Wing, M. Marcus, et al. Binge eating disorder: A multisite field trial of the diagnostic criteria *International Journal of Eating Disorders* 11 (1992): 191-203.

[3] Ecclesiastes 3:12-13.

[4] Julie Walsh. Binge-Eating That Plagues Adults Now Recognized As A Disorder *Environmental Nutrition* 11 (1997): 6.

[5] American Psychiatric Association. Diagnostic and Statistical Manual of Mental Disorders, 4th ed., text rev. (Washington D.C.: American Psychiatric Association, 2000).

Chapter 2

Is Overeating Sin?

Before we tackle the subject of overeating as sin, I want to make my motivation perfectly clear. I ache to offer you freedom, not increased guilt. But if we don't take a long hard look at overeating and what lies at its core, we will not be able to change.

Sin is an ugly word not because you are ugly. Sin is an ugly word because you are beautiful in the sight of God and your sin separates you from Him. Sin hurts us. It keeps us from realizing our destinies in Christ because in sin, we struggle to realize our full potential in knowing Him and being loved by Him. Sin looks enticing. It seems good to the eye, but just as Eve was fooled by the appearance of the forbidden fruit, we too are often fooled. At its core, sin is death. If we can understand why overeating, therefore, is a form of death, we will be in a position to move toward change.

There are four reasons why overeating is sin.

1. Negative Consequences always follow overeating.
2. Overeating expresses a lack of faith in God.
3. Overeating places food above God as an idol.
4. Overeating decreases our ability to receive from God.

NEGATIVE CONSEQUENCES ALWAYS FOLLOW OVEREATING

When a person overeats, eventually there will be physical consequences. Romans chapters 5 and 6 talk about how the outcome of sin is death and that death is the very result of sin. This death is not just spiritual death. It is also physical death. Indigestion and sleeplessness are often direct physical consequences of overeating. In addition, indirect and emergent consequences include an increased risk for obesity. This in turn can increase our risk for obesity-related diseases such as heart disease, hypertension, arthritis, cancer and diabetes.

However, the physical consequences for overeating do not stand alone. Because the soul is intricately connected to the body, it too is affected. Emotional guilt, a decrease in self-esteem and even self-abhorrence can follow overeating. These can then lead to a decline in social health as overeaters often avoid situations where they must wear formal attire or revealing garments like shorts or bathing suits. Many overeaters will not consider visiting the beach simply because they are disgusted with themselves and are ashamed to reveal their bodies in swimsuit attire. Some of my clients have sworn off parties and large dinners altogether because of their fear of overeating in front of others.

I remember a time when my family visited my aunt and uncle at their lake house. This place was an exciting getaway for a teenager to visit. We could swim all day, water ski or just lay around in the sun, talking. At the age of 15 I was deep in the trenches of bingeing and self-hate. My biggest area of concern was my hips – I hated the way they had started to expand.

Whenever we visited my aunt, she would serve food that was rarely available to me at home – chips, cookies, cold cuts, white rolls and mayonnaise. That weekend was no exception and I ate this "forbidden" food without control. The fear of weight gain ensued. Even now, over twenty years later, I remember my panic of adding to my hips that weekend. At one point, my disgust of myself was too great to bear. I decided to swim for an hour to compensate for the excessive calories. I wasn't much of a swimmer, but it was my only choice for exercise.

I swam from dock to dock, my limbs churning as if my life depended upon it. As I swam, I beat the water with my arms and legs as if I was beating myself. I quickly became exhausted, realizing I couldn't erase my fat with one long swim. I started to cry. Right there, in the water, I began to sob. My mother and aunt called out to me from a nearby dock, concerned and confused by my odd behavior. Crying and trying to stay afloat at the same time is hard to do. As I spoke to them from the water, I could barely get my words out. I was a wreck. I don't remember much after that, but I do remember my family trying to console and encourage me once I got out onto the dock. They were all so surprised with my behavior.

Yet for all their kind words, they really didn't know what to say.

It saddens me to think of the pain I've experienced most of my life regarding my eating and body image. My lack of self-acceptance hung over me like a thundercloud, preventing me from enjoying what life had to offer. In my case, overeating didn't result in obesity, but the act of bingeing itself can truly rob a person of joy and peace.

The Old Testament mentions gluttony in association with stubbornness and rebellion. The punishment actually included stoning![1] While we should be grateful the consequences for over-indulging aren't as hard today as they were in the Old Testament, we should seriously consider the behavior. God clearly does. And the repercussions for overeating are *always* negative.

OVEREATING EXPRESSES A LACK OF FAITH IN GOD.

There isn't sufficient research supporting the notion that food is physiologically addictive. Yet we can say with surety that there is an association between eating and feeling "better" emotionally. This is especially true with sugary, starchy foods as they release serotonin in the brain. Serotonin is a natural relaxation drug. This "feel good" response to food can cause a binge eater to go overboard in their portions, since almost every time a person overeats, it is in an effort to bring comfort and quell negative emotions or fears.

I believe gluttony also helps overeaters feel financially secure or protected from danger. By stockpiling supplies, we can be prepared for the unknown. By filling our stomachs with food, we are stockpiling as well. For many people, a full stomach offers feelings of security, safety, and warmth just as babies equate love and security with eating and feeding at their mother's breast. But only God Himself holds the life of every living thing in His hand. He brings forth food from the earth and supplies all living things, and both small and great look to God for their nourishment.[2]

So if a person uses food to bring about emotional satisfaction and to quiet fear and insecurity instead of having faith in God to supply all needs, is this not sin? God wants to provide us with all we need and more. We are to rely on Him with our faith for all things. Romans 14:23 says "... for whatsoever is not of faith is sin."

OVEREATING PLACES FOOD ABOVE GOD AS AN IDOL.

Another reason why overeating is sinful is found in the first commandment God gave to Moses in Exodus 20:3, "You shall have no other gods before Me." If we replace Him with anything or anyone, this replacement is idol worship.

If food gives us comfort for an emotional upset, if caffeine gives us the motivation to get up in the morning, if the second portion of dinner helps staunch anxiety over the family mealtime squabble, then we aren't allowing God to act in the place He desires to act. He wants to be involved in every detail of our lives, because He knows that nothing besides Him can bring us true happiness and deep satisfaction. But by overeating we have placed food above God. It has become our idol.

Idolatry may seem like a heavy term to apply to your second helping of pie, but it is in the small details of our every day lives that sin is so stealthy and insidious. Adding five pounds of unneeded weight in one-year tallies up to fifty pounds in ten years. And when death is knocking at our door, we wonder how we could have heart disease or Type II diabetes as believers.

God hasn't given us disease. He has given us free will and we can choose to eat and drink according to His will or outside of His will. We play a more direct role in our health than we realize. If we decide to live in obedience to Him, trusting Him for every detail of our lives, then I believe we will never gain that first five pounds to begin with and the ensuing diseases that eventually follow. God is not interested in the size of the sin (if there is such a measurement) but the heart of a person.

OVEREATING DECREASES OUR ABILITY TO RECEIVE FROM GOD.

When I first started studying my habitual binges, I considered food a curse and my desire to overeat as my greatest foe. Now I see my yearning for extra food as a blessing. When I'm most tempted to overeat, I see this desire as an indicator that something is wrong within my soul. I'm certain if you desire to binge, you are reacting to an old wound within your soul that needs healing.

If I don't heed the light on the dashboard of my car that tells me my oil is low, then I'm headed for a mechanical breakdown. This is exactly what we are doing when we stuff down emotions with excess food. If I cover up the needs of my soul with food, I'm headed for a spiritual breakdown.

When we eat to comfort ourselves, to avoid pain, to fit into a crowd, or to please someone else, we are cutting the indicator light connected to the dashboard of our emotional registry. The need for God's healing is not realized and an opportunity for change is missed. Therefore, overeating can actually stall deeper intimacy with our Creator.

This is the greatest consequence of the sin of overeating. God's perfect will is for us to walk in an intimate relationship with Him. The sin of overeating decreases our ability to enter into this kind of intimacy. Consequently, our destinies, which are completely dependent upon our level of intimacy with God, are thwarted and we cannot become all that God has called us to be.

ABSOLUTE SIN CORRUPTS ABSOLUTELY

Considering these reasons, it is clear gluttony is sin. And sin has absolute character. There is no grey area. Sin offends God first and foremost. Sin includes that second helping.

A popular Christian magazine recently featured this headline on the cover: *Why Are We So Fat? God has something to say about your lifestyle.*[3] Christians are finally waking up to the reality of this particular sin in our lives. It has quietly invaded our lives and stolen precious blessings from the people of God. Yet until we recognize it for what it is – a sin against the love of God, death at its deepest level, we cannot go another step further into healing and deliverance. However, for those who put their lives completely into God's hands (including their time at the dinner table), there is hope.

[1] Deuteronomy 21:18-2.

[2] Psalm 145:15-16.

[3] Kara Davis M.D. "Why is the Church So Fat?," *Charisma and Christian Life* June 30 (2004) cover story.

Chapter 3

Lifetime Weight Loss

The first liquid fast I accomplished lasted fourteen days. One summer, between college semesters, I found a book titled, *The Lemonade Fast* in a health food store. The recipe in the book consisted of filtered water, fresh lemon juice, maple syrup and cayenne pepper. The lemon juice and cayenne pepper cleansed my digestive system and the maple syrup gave me the energy needed to continue my daily routine. It was a simple and inexpensive fast, great for a college student on a limited budget.

This book also instructed me on the process of detoxification. It explained that after one day of fasting, my tongue would become thicker than normal and white in color. Once I had completely detoxified my body, my tongue would become clear and pink. This signaled to me that I needed to break the fast because my body had entered into starvation mode. After a couple weeks of subsisting only on lemonade, with a pink tongue to prove it, I had successfully reached my goals. I had cleansed my body, avoided all solid food and most excitingly, lost about eight pounds.

That first experience was the beginning of many lengthy fasts. I did at least two long fasts each year through my twenties and into my thirties. I was able to fast well because of my strong motivation to lose weight and lose it fast. I loved how the weight fell off, how my stomach fell flat and my skin cleared. My senses grew incredibly sharp. Even the energy experienced on a long fast, when conducted correctly, is intense. The body moves into a state of rest and all the energy used to digest food is instead transferred to normal day activities. I was even able to exercise during fasts.

There is also a feeling of euphoria that accompanies fasting. I always prayed more, read more, and pondered deeper thoughts. I felt as though I was above my normal hedonistic tendencies. After the third day of liquids, most of my regular impatience fell away. I moved slowly, thought slowly, spoke slowly. I better appreciated the present and my relationship with God always seemed deeper and more powerful.

Yet the strongest motivation supporting my fasting was that I didn't have to deal with food. I could ignore food and focus on life apart from eating. In fact, when I fasted long enough, I started to lose complete interest in food.

Over the years, I tried several different fasts and used a juicer at home to make fresh juice and broth every day. But fasting can be tricky. There is a prescribed way of starting, continuing and breaking a fast. The method used in breaking a fast is often more important than the fast itself. If you fast on liquids beyond five days and try to eat solid food without *slowly* re-introducing it to your body, you can have severe digestion problems that could last for several weeks. I had experienced both bad breaks and smooth, effortless breaks. Once I had mastered fasting, I looked forward to it as my biannual escape from my constant struggle with food.

Yet each fasting period had to end, and before plummeting to unhealthy weight levels, I had to come down out of the clouds and live on earth. This presented a colossal problem for me, since during every fast, I believed I was healed of all of my food issues. I didn't have the choice to binge during or even after fasting for at least a couple weeks (due to the importance of breaking slowly). At points during those days of liquids, I would feel like I had truly conquered my obsession with food. I was just sure in my heart there had been a deep change within me. I made promises to myself and even wrote them down in my journal: "I will never eat sugar and white, processed food again. I am free of the bondage of food. I will never gain back this weight I've lost." Inevitably, about a month after breaking my fast, I ate sugar, white processed food and gained back the weight. The pain and discouragement that followed was severe.

So why didn't fasting work for me? Because while fasting, I had believed a lie. I believed that by abstaining from all food for a season of time, I was changing my spirit and my soul. I have met other people that believe this same lie. One woman I know shared her bingeing problems with me and she felt that fasting "starved the spirit of gluttony."

Though my fasting experiences were extreme in nature compared to dieting, this same deception is analogous. We try to restrict ourselves physically, expecting spiritual change. Yet if our problem begins at a spiritual or soul level, physical restriction cannot be the solution for lifelong, permanent change.

Now let me be clear on one point – I am not against fasting. I believe there is great power in fasting and I apply it to my life regularly today. However, I did need to avoid liquid fasting for a season of time. God made it clear to me that His will for that period was "to fast from bingeing" and this was a big enough challenge for me.

WHY WE GAIN THE WEIGHT BACK

We were made for change. We are adaptive creatures and our ability to flex and bend to our environments can be likened to a chameleon. Yet most of the changes we endeavor to make are shallow and rarely last a lifetime.

Statistics tell us that 95 – 98% of all Americans that lose weight on a diet gain back the weight plus more. Even our own personal statistics support these numbers. If I were to ask you how many diets have given you *lasting* success, I would guess you could not come up with one. Yet the pull to participate in one of the latest fad diets is always present and we often fall victim to these short-term fixes regardless of our past failures.

Why do we continue to succumb? I believe part of the problem lies in our lack of understanding of how complex we are as human beings. God created us with detail and sophistication. If we were simply bodies inhabiting the planet, every diet would work and the results would bring a weight loss that would last a lifetime.

However, we are much more than physical shells. We are rational beings, existing on this earth with a spirit, soul and body.

Dr. Leslie Flynn explores the complexity of man in his book "What is Man?" and explains that "When man is viewed as no more than a body, the logical outcome is to treat people as animals. But man is worth far more than the total value of his bodily elements. Man is a unique combination of the dust of the earth and the breath of God ... What then distinguishes man from animals, if both are living creatures or living souls? It is this – when God breathed into man's nostrils the breath of life, He created a part of man in His own divine image."[1]

By appreciating our identities as complex images of God Himself, we are better able to understand why we do what we do, and why we don't do what we should.

"Spirit, soul and body are connected and affect one another."

This principle is part of the backbone for true, lasting change. In order to understand the importance of this principle, we must first study ourselves as triune beings.

I am indebted to Reverend Dutch Sheets for his course *Becoming Who You Are, the Theology of the Soul*.[2] Through his teaching, I became aware of the complexity of my makeup and the process by which I live. The following are his definitions of the different parts of our identities.

SPIRIT — This is the part of us that can relate to God. It includes our conscience and intuition. Our spirit distinguishes us from the animal world. As Christians our spirits have been reborn[3] and we are new.[4] This takes place instantly the moment we ask Jesus to save us from ourselves, our history and the path of destruction we are on without Him.

SOUL — The soul is the part of us that relates to our world around us. The soul is made up of our **mind, will** and **emotions**. This part of us is unregenerate, with its natural bend toward sin. Once we are born again, God begins a process of renewal in our souls and this process will continue until the day we die.[5]

The soul also holds our memory and subconscious mind. 85 – 90% of the decisions we make are based upon our memories and subconscious mind,[6] so this part of the soul is an extremely important aspect to consider when we try to bring about lifetime change.

"As the seat of our identity and will, the soul functions as the command center of the human being. What goes on there determines the extent to which the King's rule will be manifest in the whole of our being. If there is brokenness or malfunction there, it may not mean my damnation, but it does cause the Holy Spirit consternation." Jack Hayford, "Rebuilding the Real You."[7]

BODY — Our bodies are the outer shells that respond to the decisions of the soul. Matthew Henry describes the body as "frail, mortal ... it is a house of clay, whose foundation is in the dust. The life purchased and promised does not immortalize the body in its present state. It is dead ... "[8]

FLESH — Our identity is made up of three parts but the flesh, which is part of the soul, is important to review if we are going to understand our behaviors. The New Strong's Exhaustive Concordance definition for flesh includes, "... the infirmity of human nature;[9] the corrupt nature of man subject to the filthy appetites and passions;[10] in regard to our present weak and corruptible state."[11]

The flesh belongs to the lower or unregenerate region of man's being. Jack Hayford explains it this way, "Bondages such as fear, anger, bitterness, lust ... etc. are lodged in the area of your soul, not your spirit. This can be clearly seen if we pause to consider how all of these involve our mind (how we think), our emotions (how we feel), and our will (how we act)."[12] They are not in your spirit because of the rebirth in Jesus. But the body and soul are still in process.

There are scriptures that refer to the whole person consisting of all three parts such as 1 Thessalonians 5:23, "Now may the God of peace Himself sanctify you completely; and may your whole spirit, soul and body be preserved blameless at the coming of our Lord Jesus Christ," and Mark 12:30, "The first of all the commandments is: 'Hear, O Israel, the LORD our God, the LORD is one. And you shall love the Lord your God with all your heart, with all your soul, with all your mind, and with all your strength.'"

Though spirit, soul and body are connected, we can also see a differentiation between them. Hebrews 4:12 states "For the word of God is living and powerful, and sharper than any two-edged sword, piercing even to the division of soul and spirit." Here we see that there is a difference between soul and spirit and that the word of God actually divides the two, making their unique distinctions clear.

Christianity is one of the only religions teaching that the three parts of man's identity (spirit, soul, and body) are interconnected. Many other world religions treat the body as unimportant and disconnected from the spirit and soul.[13] With this kind of mindset, sin committed by the body is often rationalized as inconsequential in regard to one's position with God. Yet Christianity strongly refutes this position throughout its doctrine.

Christ Himself took on flesh and blood, demonstrating the value of the body and our connection to Him exists because He had a human soul and body while he walked this earth. His walk on earth was sinless in spirit, soul and body and because of this; He was able to stand as the sacrificial lamb on our behalf. We can experience supernatural healing because of Christ's body. The scriptures say that He was bruised for our transgressions and that by the stripes on His back we are healed. Our very salvation leans upon the physical body of Jesus Christ. His resurrection was not only of His spirit, but also of His physical body. Even in the ages to come we will be given a new, physical earth and will reign over it with transformed physical bodies.

Medical doctors and recent research are continually supporting the strong link between spirit, soul and body. Disease is often traced back to spiritual problems such as unresolved guilt, anger or unforgiveness. Hypertension, arthritis, ulcers and even cancer are diseases that have been connected to spiritual and emotional dilemmas.[14,15]

There are several depictions in scripture that note this association between spirit, soul and body.

Proverbs is replete with examples. Before reading these verses, note that the bones are the source of supply of blood for the body and our marrow is also the area of the body responsible for our immune system. All of disease is fought based on the health of our bones.

Proverbs 3:7-8, "Do not be wise in your own eyes; fear the Lord and turn away from evil. It will be healing to your body and refreshment to your bones." (NAS)

Proverbs 14: 30, "A sound heart is life to the body, but envy is rottenness to the bones."

Proverbs 15:30, "The light of the eyes rejoices the heart, and a good report makes the bones healthy."

Proverbs 17:22, "A merry heart does good, like medicine, but a broken spirit dries the bones."

Additionally, the Word of God is offered as medicine for the body in many places. Consider Proverbs 4:20-22, "My son, give attention to my words; incline your ear to my sayings. Do not let them depart from your eyes; keep them in the midst of your heart; for they are life to those who find them, and health to all their flesh."

With this understanding of the interconnection of spirit, soul and body, every negative or positive behavior performed by the body must be understood as an expression of the soul and spirit. Any health program that focuses upon the body alone (including some fasts) as a separate, indifferent part of a person offers only temporary, shallow results. The spirit, soul and body are to be inextricably included and considered in all decisions made for change. The root of every behavior originates in the soul and unless this origin is uncovered and understood, the changes sought for a lifetime will only last for a day.

---

[1] Leslie B. Flynn. *Man: Ruined and Restored* (Wheaton, IL: Victor Books, 1978), 16,17.

[2] Rev. Dutch Sheets. *Becoming Who You Are: Course Study Guide* (Columbus, GA: Christian Life School of Theology), 2-8.

[3] 1 Peter 1:23.

[4] 2 Corinthians 5:17.

[5] Ephesians 1:1, Ephesians 4:17-32, 2 Corinthians 3:18, Romans 12:1-2.

[6] Rev. Dutch Sheets. *Becoming Who You Are: Course Study Guide* (Columbus, GA: Christian Life School of Theology), 6-8.

[7] Jack W. Hayford. *Rebuilding the Real You* (Ventura, CA: Regal Books, 1986), 60.

[8] Matthew Henry. *Matthew Henry's Commentary on the Bible* (Peabody, MA: Hendrickson Publishers, 1997), Romans 8:10.

[9] James Strong. *The New Exhaustive Concordance of the Bible* (Nashville, TN: Thomas Nelson Publisher's, 1995), Hebrews 5:7.

[10] James Strong. *The New Exhaustive Concordance of the Bible* (Nashville, TN: Thomas Nelson Publisher's, 1995), John 3:6, Romans 7:18, 7:25, 8:16, Galatians 5:13, 16, 19, 6:8.

[11] James Strong. *The New Exhaustive Concordance of the Bible* (Nashville, TN: Thomas Nelson Publisher's, 1995), Matthew 16:17, Galatians 1:6, Ephesians 6:12.

[12] Jack Hayford. *Cleansing Stream Seminar Workbook, Session One: Alignment* (Northridge, CA: Glory Communications, 1995), 21.

[13] One of the basic concepts of Eastern thought is the concept of material illusion (maya in Hindu); the material world is an illusion, and sin is nothing but ignorance about the fact of illusion. Josh McDowell and Don Stewart. *Answers To Tough Questions: What Skeptics Are Asking About The Christian Faith* (Nashville, TN: Thomas Nelson, 1993), 116.

[14] S.I. McMillen M.D. and David E. Stern M.D. *None of These Diseases The Bible's Health Secrets For The 21st Century* 3rd edition (Grand Rapids, MI: Fleming H. Revell, 2000), 167-177.

[15] Art Mathias. *In His Own Image* (Anchorage, AL: Wellspring Publishing, 2003), 29,31-73,166-167, 201-202,123-133.

The Process of Lasting Change

The increase of appetite grows by what it feeds on.

A pudgy Italian pastor used this phrase in a sermon one time. He explained that he loved pasta and the more he consumed, the more his love for it increased. This principle applies to all areas of our lives. The more familiar a food, a behavior, a thought process, the more attracted to it we become. How do we make sure that we increase our "feeding" on healthful choices?

The answer lies in the process by which we make decisions. Once we have accepted Jesus as our Lord and Savior, our spirits are subject to the Holy Spirit. This is what causes us to "do right." The flesh is our weakness and it presses us to "do wrong." The soul, though unregenerate, can be pulled by the flesh or spirit in either direction. Every day we experience a battle as these two parts fight for dominance of the soul. The decisions made by the soul are then expressed in the body. (See illustration, next page.)

Here's an example of this process in exercise. In pursuit of a stronger heart, lungs, and muscles, I may plan to go out for a twenty-minute run. I've run this distance before and I know I am capable. When I start the run, in the initial six minutes, I experience the first stage of aerobic exercise. It is uncomfortable. I have pain in my muscles, my heart is stressed, and my lungs can't seem to take in enough air. Both my flesh and spirit acknowledge these signals. Yet which one will control the response?

With my flesh in command of my soul, I may process these physiological signs as good reason to stop running. The flesh always wants the easy way out. It always looks for shortcuts and the path of least resistance. The flesh is weak and it will direct you into weak decisions that will lead to a weak existence.

Meanwhile, since the soul is still going through the process of regeneration, it is already leaning toward weakness. It doesn't take

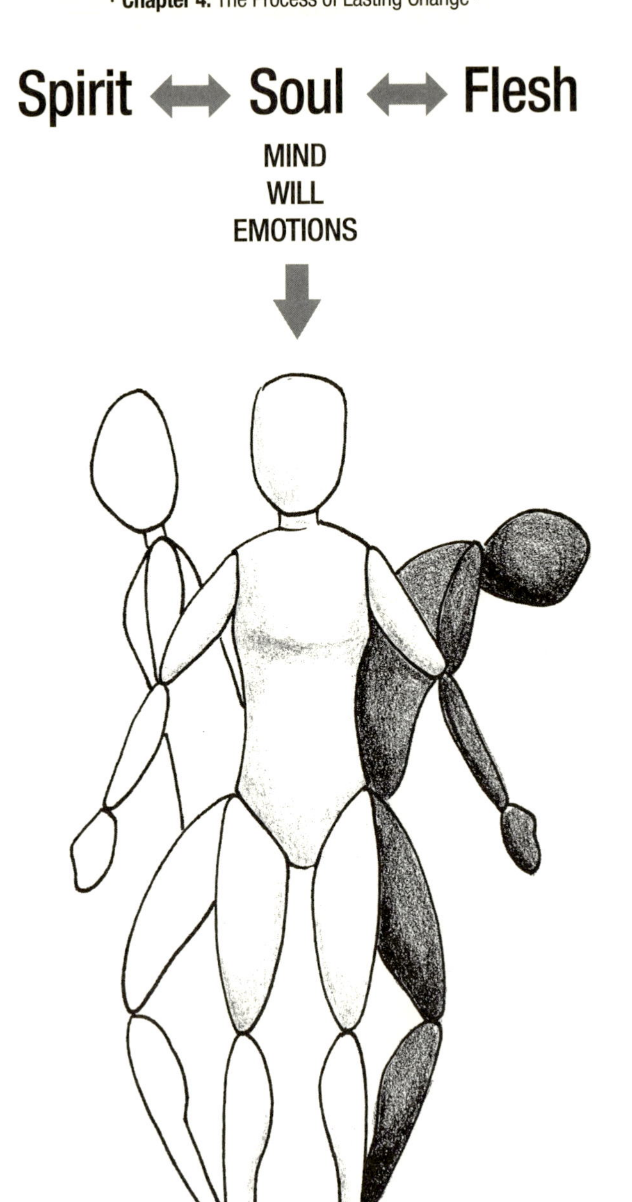

Behavior Expressed in My Body

much to tip the scale in the wrong direction. Jesus said "Watch and pray, that you enter not into temptation: the spirit indeed is willing but the flesh is weak."[1]

Mike Bickle, author and founder of the International House of Prayer in Kansas City, MO, has devoted over ten years of study and research to the book in the Bible known as Song of Songs, or Song of Solomon. His study helped me understand the power of this verse.[2] Though Jesus pointed out that the flesh is weak, he notes the willing spirit within us. He sees that our heart's desire is to draw nearer to Him and to do what is pleasing to Him. Though I may struggle with exercise and discomfort, the Holy Spirit can lead me to strength. It is a supernatural occurrence. We can do nothing apart from this strength[3] and we can do everything He calls us to do with this strength.[4] All it takes is a willing spirit, and everyone that loves Jesus has this willing spirit.

With my spirit in command of my soul, we can see the discomfort in the first few minutes of exercise as part of the process of change. I can welcome it as a temporary experience, having the faith that I will soon get past those initial stages of discomfort and come into a more comfortable place as I run beyond six minutes. The success of my completed run is dependent upon how I process the physical stimulants – by my flesh or by my spirit.[5]

So not only are spirit, soul and body connected, there is a specific order that is best to follow. *When my spirit governs my soul and my soul governs my body, there is lasting change.* However, many of us live in the opposite direction. The world has fed us the lie that if we focus on our bodies changing, our souls and spirits will follow. Par for the course, the world always turns the truths of God upside down.

The truth is that *the body plays a very limited role in our health.* I have heard many say that their bodies have minds of their own and that they have to fight the cravings of their bodies. This is an inaccurate perception. The body certainly gives us hunger pains, discomfort while exercising and feelings of fatigue when we do not get enough rest. Yet these signals are processed by the soul first before subsequent behavior by the body is made. And with the spirit in control, the soul is subject to its power as the spirit is subject to the Holy Spirit. Most programs and diets place too much emphasis on the body and too little on the other parts of our identity.

LIFE TREE MODEL

A model I use to explain the dynamics in human behavior is a Life Tree. The fruit of the tree are the behaviors that we see evident in our lives. Galatians 5 lists the fruit of the flesh and the fruit of the spirit. The trunk of the tree represents our lifestyles and habits and the roots of the tree represent values, attitudes and beliefs. (See illustration, opposite page.)

If I see bad fruit at the top of my tree, cutting the bad fruit off will not solve my problem. With the same roots, trunk and branches remaining, I will yield the same fruit again during the "next harvest." It's the same with diets and most quick fix programs. The issue lies in the roots of a person, not the fruit itself. The fruit is only an outward sign of an inward problem. I will return to this Life Tree model throughout the book. For now, you only need to know that the solution to your bad behavior is "root deep."

In working with clients who desire weight loss, men are usually less aware of the deeper, root reasons for their overeating. They simply aren't as in touch with their feelings and therefore have trouble connecting their overeating with the unmet needs of their souls.

One of my clients often challenged me in this area. He could not make the connection between his binges and his emotions. He often said to me, "I don't overeat because I am upset. I just eat because I love food."

Though "love" is a term overused in our society today, I always take notice when a person refers to food with love. To delight in food is one thing, but to think about it throughout the day, make great efforts to attain it and then dive into it at mealtime as though it is the last piece of indulgence on earth, causes me to consider if it has taken on the form of what Jack Frost calls a "counterfeit affection."[6] Frost is the author of the book, *Experiencing the Father's Embrace,* and his teaching on the love of Father God has penetrated nations suffering from what he calls an "orphan spirit." He explains in his book that

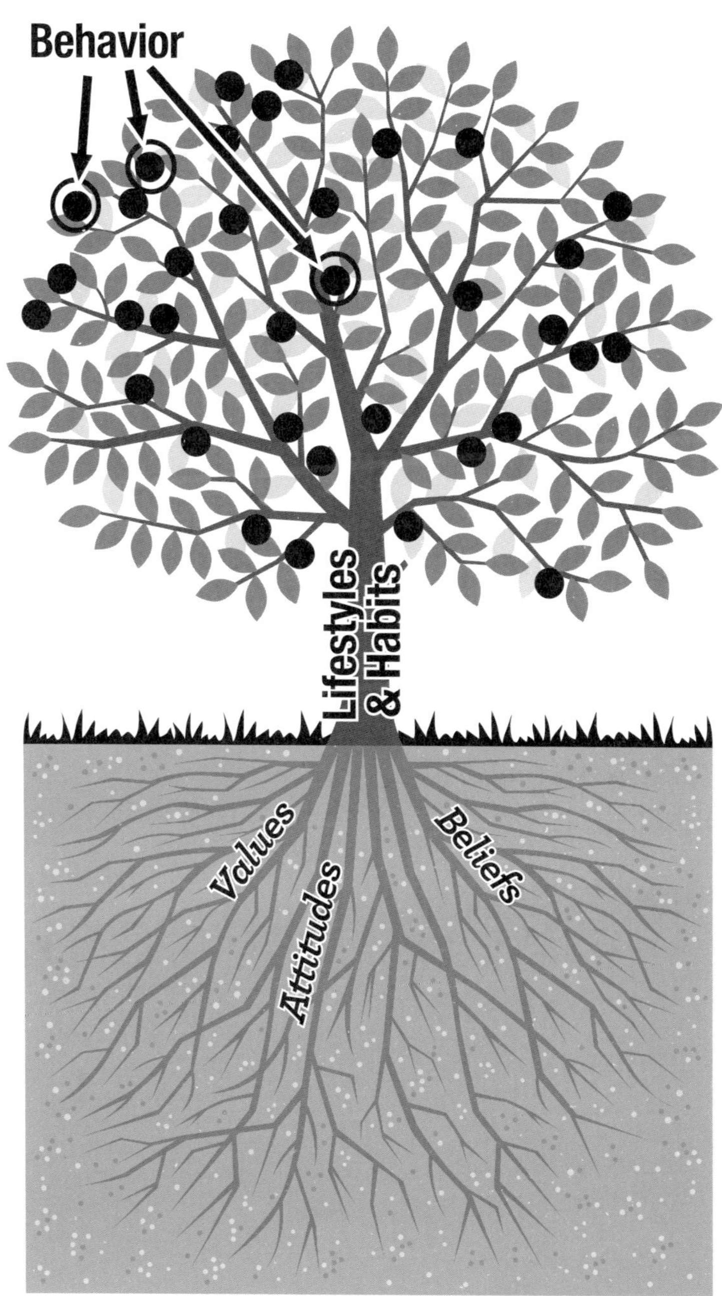
Behavior
Lifestyles & Habits
Values
Attitudes
Beliefs

when we are disconnected to the Father's love, we turn to these imitations instead, living like orphans instead of children of God. Though temporary and faulty and only a mock for God's solution, it is a solution nonetheless and oftentimes, it is the easier solution to choose.

When we begin to see our desire for extra food as a signal that we have problematic issues in our "roots," then we can allow Him to address our need. Without this realization of the interconnectedness of our spirit, soul and body, we have trouble identifying our need for God and therefore, our bad fruit doesn't change. Worse yet, the growth of our relationship with God becomes stagnant.

The purpose of this chapter, and the rest of this book for that matter, is to offer freedom. Where the spirit of the Lord is, there is freedom.[7] Freedom from disease, bondage, and the power of the flesh dominating the decisions of the soul. We only realize and enjoy this freedom when we begin to look at the entire picture of who we are and why we live as we do. I have found freedom from the bondage of food addiction. Now I offer it to you.

---

[1] Matthew 26:41.

[2] Mike Bickle. *Song of Songs. The Ravished Heart of God with Mike Bickle* (Kansas City, MO: Friends of the Bridegroom, 1999), Session 6, 1-6.

[3] John 15:5.

[4] Philippians 4:13.

[5] Romans 8:5-13.

[6] Jack Frost. *Experiencing the Father's Embrace* (Lake Mary, FL: Charisma House, 2002), 63.

[7] 2 Corinthians 3:17.

Chapter 5

Does Your History Define You?

Self-Modification and the theory of behavior change have been used to bring about change in people's lives since the dawn of psychology. In my life, I found freedom from negative behavior by applying some of the basic principles of self-modification.

In applying these principles, I have, however, challenged them with the word of God and either agree with or refute their relevance for the Christian believer.

ANTECEDENTS — these are the stimulants or triggers in our lives that cause us to respond.[1] Antecedents can be sights, smells, sounds - anything our senses can register. They can be people or things people say. Yet antecedents don't have to go through one of our five senses to affect us. They can also be fed to us through our minds by Satan's lies or by God's truth spoken to us through the Holy Spirit. In Genesis 3 we see a clear example of how Satan spoke to Eve as he enticed her to eat from the forbidden tree. We can also see how God speaks through the Holy Spirit on several occasions. One example is found in the thirteenth chapter of the book of Acts when the disciples were instructed specifically by God, through the Holy Spirit, to send out Barnabas and Saul for evangelism. (There are many more examples of such and promises found in the Bible that tell us that God desires and is able to speak clearly to us regarding all situations.)[2]

Once an antecedent makes contact with us, we process this contact and follow it with a way of thinking. Then, at some point, we behave in a way that responds to our thinking. Our thought - life is in fact the birthplace for all behavior, just as the roots of a tree are the source of life for the fruit. The Bible speaks of the power and importance of our thinking.[3]

QUALITIES OF ANTECEDENTS — One important quality of an antecedent is that it is attached to a **history** somewhere within our past experiences. Often the behaviors we live out today are products of the early history of our lives, evolving around our childhood, our growing up years, when we were most impressionable. At that time, we were surrounded by situations, stimulants. We responded to these stimulants, perhaps in different ways at first, but then settled upon one way to respond and this then formed habits, which now can orchestrate our lives in the present.

The same antecedent can affect two people very differently based upon their histories with the antecedent. The smell of popcorn, for example. Let's say a person was brought up in a family that often went to the movies for entertainment. And whenever this family went to the movies, they ate popcorn. Over time, popcorn and family fun became strongly connected. Therefore, when this person smells fresh popcorn, the combination of the desire to eat it and experience that connection to family again may entice him to overindulge.

If, on the other hand, a person was left home by parents to make dinner without help or companionship and if microwave popcorn was the old standby, a connection between popcorn and loneliness might have occurred. The connection would still be strong but quite negative and so this person may have an overwhelming distaste for popcorn and will avoid it at all costs. Thus, the same exact antecedent can bring about two different reactions based upon the history of the antecedent.

BEHAVIOR — In this context, when we talk about behavior, we are referring to responses to antecedents.[4] As Christians, our behaviors are dependent upon two effects:

1. Our history and
2. Our place of deliverance concerning our history.

The first effect, our history, is registered in our souls. Remember, our souls include our mind, will and emotions. All that has ever happened to us is stored in our minds as memories. These memories can be conscious or subconscious. It is believed that 85 – 90% of our behavior is controlled by our subconscious mind. Yet the power in our subconscious mind lies unrealized. In considering food, we may think that our conscious mind has the power to decrease our intake of sweets, but in reality, our history, stored in our subconscious, has much more influence upon our eating.

You may think you're just a dessert freak and you have always had a sweet tooth. But the history of this belief pattern may include the fact that your Mom always served dessert after dinner and didn't accept rejection of her desserts very well. Perhaps rejecting her homemade apple pie was taken personally and therefore, you have learned, at a deep level, that eating dessert after dinner is the right thing to do (in order to stay in your mother's graces). You may not be aware of these details in your conscious mind but they play a powerful role in your present day decisions.

I experienced this power in a dramatic way when flying from Seattle, WA to Tokyo, Japan. One of the engines in our plane caught fire and we were forced to turn around and make an emergency landing abruptly on the airport runway. We popped all of the 747's tires and were then rushed out of the plane, onto the yellow blow-up escape route (the one pictured in your emergency landing pamphlet) and told to run to a nearby field in case the plane blew up. All went well, the plane did not catch fire and the next day we boarded a second plane to Tokyo. That flight was without consequence and I experienced no fear whatsoever. Yet unexpectedly, two months later, my subconscious mind caught up with my conscious mind and when I boarded a plane to Korea for a short visit, I began to break a sweat, my entire body trembling. Try as I might, I could not calm down.

I had never had any fear of flying before this emergency landing. Yet now, starting with my trip to Korea, I could barely make it through takeoff and landing. It took me two years to re-adjust to flying.

In the same way that I was impacted by that one event, we are greatly affected by events that took place in our past. Our subconscious mind can "hide" the results until a subsequent, familiar event comes along. Then we are surprisingly controlled by that past event in our present day behaviors. It is imperative for us to understand the power of the past and the connection between antecedents and behavior in order to allow God to break us from bondage to old events and the negative behavior that soon follows, in this case, overeating.

HISTORY is powerful in our lives in the present-time because of two qualities — **1. Repetition, 2. High impact/association with emotions.**

Not only was it **repetitive**, (Mom made dessert after dinner each night, I ate dessert after dinner each night), but it was also **highly impacting** (Mom would get upset if I did not eat dessert and would take it as rejection) and **strongly associated with emotions** (when I ate dessert after dinner, I felt loved. When I didn't eat dessert I felt sad and rejected for my decision. I also felt guilty).

Both parts do not need to be present for a strong connection in history to be created. I can be verbally abused by someone one time (no repetition) and have it affect me for life because of the high impact and the emotion associated with the situation. I can also experience a repetitive association without emotion or high impact and yet the repetition itself can create the strength of the A/B Association (Antecedent/Behavior Association).

There was a period in which I drank coffee with a piece of fruit every morning. I enjoyed this combination for several months. One afternoon I began eating a grapefruit for a mid-afternoon snack and I found myself longing for a cup of coffee. I thought to myself, "That's strange. I never drink coffee in the afternoon and I have no need for a caffeine boost today. Why do I yearn for coffee right now?" Then it struck me that the grapefruit had linked me to my morning routine of fruit and coffee and therefore the urge for a cup of java followed. Again that Italian pastor comes to mind and the principle that says,

The increase of appetite grows by what it feeds on.

These kinds of connections can be very strong. And they can form mindsets, belief patterns, and then habits or patterns of behavior and even cultural structures and eventually the general health of a cultural group or nation. In Christian language, these are called strongholds.

We can witness these associations in people we know, including our own selves. Let's look at some examples of antecedents and behaviors that are based solely upon a person's history:

"I have never been a morning person and I never will be."

The history of this belief pattern may be –

"All my life I hated getting up in the morning because I hated school and never wanted to go."

Or, "Exercise and I just don't mix."

The history of this belief pattern may be –

"I barely passed gym class and I was always the last kid to get picked for the teams."

The association between an antecedent and our following beliefs and consequential behavior is based strongly upon our history. This is an A/B Association.

If our lives were only dictated by our history, we would be a sorry lot. Thank God our behaviors are based upon TWO effects:
1. Our history **and**
2. Our place of deliverance concerning our history.

The first part, our connection to our history, is strong, and for all the world, insurmountable and impossible to change truly at a deep level. But the second part, our place of deliverance in Christ, can save us from our natural response.

We can experience deliverance and inward change so that our past does not have to orchestrate our present any longer! Is that hard to believe?

If we keep in mind that, *spirit, soul and body are connected and affect one another,* we can believe it because our behavior is based upon whether we are living according to our spirit or our flesh. Remembering ***the increase of appetite grows by what it feeds on,*** we can tip the scales in favor of our spirits when we feed our spirits and starve our flesh. So how do we do this? Read on and find out.

---

[1] David L. Watson and Roland G. Tharp. *Self-Directed Behavior Self-Modification for Personal Adjustment* (Belmont, CA: Wadsworth Publishing, 1997), 10-13, 123-125.

[2] John 16:13, Luke 21:12-15, Acts 13:1-4, 1 Corinthians 14:6-33.

[3] James 3:14-15, Eph. 4:17-24, 2 Corinthians 10:3-5.

[4] David L. Watson and Roland G. Tharp. *Self-Directed Behavior Self-Modification for Personal Adjustment* (Belmont, CA: Wadsworth Publishing, 1997), 10-13.

· Chapter 6 ·

God Knows Best

STEP 1: Release our methods of change for God's method

While cutting hefty slices of chocolate birthday cake at a party, my friends asked me a familiar question, "How many calories are there in each piece?" These friends of mine seemed to always be on a diet of some sort and having a notion of what I do for a living, I was the perfect source of information.

I thought about the type of cake and icing; included the large scoop of ice cream accompanying it, and calculated the damage in my mind. "About 600 or so."

The groans of fear escaped the mouths of my friends as they contemplated the consequences of their upcoming indulgence. I took a bite of cake, enjoying its sweet taste and moist texture.

"A piece of birthday cake is not a problem ... unless you have it tomorrow night and the night after that," I said. I took another bite of cake, and watched their reactions. I could tell by their expressions that they did not understand my logic. As far as they were concerned, they were about to blow it. With this one portion of cake and ice cream, any diet that was on active duty would soon be aborted. I could almost read their minds. I too had thought the same things when enjoying high calorie food: Wave goodbye to a smaller waistline ... so long to my summer bathing suit dreams ... it's all over now, may as well give in and stop trying ... it just isn't worth it.

"Extreme thinking" such as the above example is popular with dieters. However, it isn't part of God's plan for your health. A sapling takes a lifetime to reach maturity. Likewise, most of our important life achievements take time as well. Weight loss and health improvement are no different. If a person's weight drops drastically over a short period, it usually occurs by a method contrary to God's plan for health. He created our physical bodies with intricate detail and they can adapt quickly to extreme change, but our souls (the source of our mind, will and emotions), as the more controlling force, can only change through a process of slow, consistent steps.

So herein lies our first challenge when trying to alter a behavior pattern . . . surrendering our own methods of weight loss in order to hear and respond to God's method of change. In all areas of life, we must release our mindset for His mindset, our timing for His timing, and our agenda for His agenda; diet and exercise included.

Prior to knowing this, I had always dealt with weight gain by dieting, fasting or exercising in extreme amounts. These methods offered temporary life style changes, which brought about quick results. It also gave me a sense of control. But the truth is, I was consistently out of control and I was ignoring the need for deeper work in my soul.

While this method can be very enticing, it is merely surface work. There is little pain or inner reflection. When we engage in quick fix programs that do not address the roots of our behaviors, it is like placing a small bandage over a deep heart wound that needs intensive surgery.

In addition, quick, temporary change is a major deception in our culture today. You only have to tune into the vast plethora of media advertisements offering instant change to see the lie in play. One actor on a recent cell phone commercial admits, "I want to feel like I can get virtually everything for virtually nothing." Another says, "I want to feel like I'm not limited by time, space ... " Our natural, carnal nature is always enticed to view solutions from a temporary, worldly perspective and not with a heavenly, eternal mindset. Yet the truth illustrated in the Bible is that "We do not wrestle against flesh and blood, but against principalities, against powers, against the rulers of the darkness of this age."[1] Though this verse may conjure up images of demon powers, I think there is more to it than that for we can find these negative influences within our very own mindsets.

The word **principalities** in the Greek means the origin of something, the beginning of something. Think of the first time your relationship with food changed from normal to abnormal. When did you feel you had to fight with food as though it had power you couldn't ignore? This perspective of food had a beginning in your life. It is crucial that you trace back to this time in order to understand your present obsession with food. When you first began thinking and using food outside of the roles of nutrition and celebration, a principality took root in your soul. It may have found its starting place in your thinking the first time your mother told you not to eat candy because girls aren't allowed to enjoy sweet food. Perhaps it came later in life, when you gave birth to your first child and you couldn't lose your "baby fat" for years afterward.

I gained my first unacceptable five pounds at age thirteen. While visiting my aunt and uncle in Illinois, I worked at their public pool, in the snack shop. Naturally during breaks I indulged in the same fries and ice cream I sold to customers. I'm sure I was nervous and at times, uncomfortable, since I was living away from home, so I found comfort in the food around me. The weight gain was fast. When I returned home, my Mom put me on my first strict diet and I lost those five pounds in a hurry. It is important to note that the deeper issue at work in that first diet was the fear in my mom that I would have weight problems all of my life. She had struggled with her weight as well and her disdain for my weight gain only passed on her fears to me. Thus I was introduced to the **principality** of weight gain/weight loss and the struggle with food as enemy.

Next, when fully rooted, these principalities become powers in our lives that dominate our thoughts and actions. The word **powers** in the Greek speaks of domain, jurisdiction, what is permitted and permissible. Though we may reject these mindsets at first, they soon are permitted to rule in a few cases, then subsequently more often until finally they become innately second nature to us. My first abuse of food in Illinois, the five-pound gain and subsequent crash diet could have been a onetime event, but I continued misusing food all through high school as I gained five pounds every weekend and then lost it by skipping breakfast and lunch Monday through Friday. Because I was so entrenched in this cycle, these behaviors gained strength and my struggle with food began to truly become a domain, a **power** in my life.

Finally, the word **rulers** in this context means world rule, the ruler of this world. This part of the process denotes a final acceptance and ultimately submission to the way of the world, even though it is counter to God's plan for our lives. In regard to food, I

Diet Mindset

The Issue	Diet Mindset
1. Focus	Focus is on the body alone
2. Process	Drastic changes and drastic weight loss in a short amount of time
3. Thought-Life	Negative thinking, all or nothing, extreme changes, peaks and valleys
4. Discomfort	Hated and avoided as something negative
5. Food	Live to eat, obsessed with food; hold a grudge over food
6. Exercise	Used to get the weight off; Immediate and full-time commitment
7. Forbidden Foods	Avoid completely, fear, considered illegal, morally bad; addicted to
8. Rest	What rest?; lack of boundaries
9. Success	Desired Goal Weight, Exercise Adherence, "Perfect" Eating
10. Overall Perception	Perfectionistic, impatient, difficulty accepting the present

consider the way of the world, or the ruler, to be the diet mindset and all it entails. Following is a chart I use to compare a healthy mindset with the diet mindset.

vs. Healthy Mindset

Healthy Mindset

Focus is on the spirit, soul and body,
considering them as connected and affecting one another

Step by step changes are made in lifestyle,
while including the roots of all behavior – mindsets and perceptions of life, self, others and God

Moderation, steady flying, constant string of hope pervades every aspect of life

Understood as necessary and embraced as part of the process of change

Eat to Live, at peace with food, eat for sustenance, celebration and enjoyment

Used to increase self-esteem, endorphins, energy and mental acuity; Slowly introduced with moderation

Gradually re-introduce into food plan with moderation and control; you control food, no addiction

Essential, planned & protected with boundaries

Increased intimacy with God, peace with self and food, increased energy, health and body confidence,
body stays comfortably in its natural weight

Observing, revealing, flexible, forgiving, changing, accepting the present with hope for the future

Consider the following list of diet habits to see if you have fallen prey to the world's method of weight loss:

1. Drink two glasses of water before every meal (in actuality, research has shown that water intake encourages food intake)[2]
2. Eat vegetables at home before going to a party
3. Use only small plates
4. Eat only when sitting down at the table (with lighted candles!)
5. Eat only half of what is on your plate
6. Avoid all white foods (sugar, flour, potatoes)
7. Eat raw foods to increase the calories burned in digestion
8. Never eat after 9:00 p.m.
9. Chew each bite twenty times before swallowing
10. Don't snack between meals (we now know that small snacks between meals decrease overeating in meals and keeps the metabolism at peak efficiency)

Delores struggled with a diet mindset for months before we came to a breakthrough in her eating. She had tasted success from dropping weight almost effortlessly on strict diets only to eventually gain it all back. As we met together, I explained to her that she would have to stop all dieting in order to begin eating God's way; to find peace with her food and body. For weeks she struggled with coming to this place of submission in her heart where she could adopt God's plan for her health.

One day Delores arrived at an appointment and as soon as we finished our starting prayer she said to me, "I have come to barter with you and get your permission to go on an 'induction diet' for just two weeks." Even as she asked me this, I felt the Lord saying to me, "Don't budge." I smiled and said that I could not agree with her two-week diet plan. By caving in, I would be agreeing to yet another period of deprivation and the disappointment that would surely come as the weight returned after her two weeks of dieting ended.

She responded with frustration. She hated herself and wanted her extra weight off as soon as possible. She was desperate because she realized her weight loss goal for Christmas was unattainable.

I asked her, "Is it your goal or God's goal?" I then explained that she had to see herself as loved by God in that moment before God could really do a work in her life.

She winced at the thought of accepting His love in her present condition. Her clothes didn't fit, her digestion was messed up and the holidays were right around the corner.

When thinking back on my years of bulimia and binge eating, giving up my method of "extreme living" for God's method of "moderation in all things" didn't interest me one bit. I was all about drama. Though I was not the rebellious type, I had discovered by my early teens that my own ways of gaining attention from friends and family worked. My opinions were strong, my arguments forceful, my emotions erratic, my exercise excessive and the latest diet craze I engaged in was always severe. If I wasn't a vegetarian, I was fasting on liquids, if I wasn't fasting on liquids, I was avoiding all sugar and flour, and the pattern continued on and on.

I believe now that I was as addicted to the lows of my drama-queen life as I was to the highs. At least while dwelling on negative thoughts about my body, I could obsess about the next exciting new diet I was going to use for quick weight loss, and the emotional high from attacking another challenge. This addiction to radical, fast weight loss and the inevitable weight gain defined me as a person. My life revolved around my relationship with food.

I also enjoyed fantasy thoughts about my physical image. I often visualized a thinner me as I would stare at the images on television or in glamour magazines. I would fixate on the bodies Hollywood and society regularly applauded. In a compulsive fashion I found myself repeating goals for weight loss: "Just ten pounds, just ten pounds, I need to lose ten pounds." My desire for a perfect body was so deeply entrenched in my mindset that mantras like this were commonplace and never questioned.

Often connected to these thoughts were daydreams about intimacy with a future husband, a perfect home and perfect children. I thought this way for so long that I started believing I wouldn't have a husband, a home or children until I was perfectly thin.

I even thought success in my career was dependent upon my relationship with food. I can remember marveling at the men and women who succeeded in their relationships and careers while still being overweight. Being overweight was not an option for me. I believed I had to be thin and successful – or overweight and unsuccessful.

At age twenty-two, I was suffering from clinical depression. I tried to let go of my food addiction, but the thought of doing so scared me. I once wrote in my journal,

> *"Today I realized that without food as my center, my life as I have built it thus far is not captivating, not exciting, not me. As I'm letting go of food as my center, my reason for living, the true bones of Heidi are really quite boring…"*

That was a sad realization for me, but coming to terms with myself was a significant part of the change that followed.

I see now that I was not physically addicted to food, but addicted to the saga I had created around the food in my life. I didn't know this at the time, but my obsession with food allowed me to ignore deeper fears like rejection, loneliness, and failure. I will cover this with more detail in following chapters. For now it is important to note that we look to quick fix solutions in order to avoid the deeper, harder issues of life.

Don't we all hunger for the quick fix solution without personal effort? Look again at this wish from the T.V. commercial, "I want to feel like I'm not limited by time, space. ..." The truth is we are limited in this life by time and space. Changing our old mindsets of health, body, food and exercise will be painstakingly slow. Yet we must move slowly. This is the **only** way to permanent change.

Lifetime change occurs
through a process of small steps.

Julia Cameron, a writer for writers, states in, *The Artist's Way*, her explanation of the process of creative recovery. She explains, "Too far, too fast, and we can undo ourselves. Creative recovery is like marathon training. We want to log ten slow miles for every one fast mile. This can go against the ego's grain. We want to be great – immediately great – but that is not how recovery works. It is an awkward, tentative, even embarrassing process. There will be many times when we won't look good – to ourselves or anyone else. We need to stop demanding that we do. It is impossible to get better and look good at the same time."[3]

Once we begin the journey towards health and wholeness, we must see it much like training for a marathon. It requires a long-term commitment. It will demand patience and diligence.

Perhaps in dropping the diet practices you have held for so long, you will initially gain weight. This has happened to a few of my clients.

Once Delores started releasing restrictive diets and extreme change, she came to me, panicked. She was gaining weight instead of losing it. But she had other issues to deal with too. She had been on a very strict diet prior to meeting with me. Her health was poor due to the restrictions of the diet, and she was also in desperate need of repair in her soul. We started working on her relationship with God and releasing her diet to the Lord. As the reality of her fears and insecurities came to the surface, the weight gain came as well. "This isn't me! I am not fat like this. I don't have a tummy that makes me look pregnant!"

"Maybe this is you," I said gently. "Maybe your body, for the first time in years, is finally allowed to express who you really are on the inside. Maybe this heavier you has been there all along, but you never wanted to look at her. Only after you look at the truth of where you are spiritually, emotionally, and physically, can you get the healing you need for change."

THEN GOD

I related well to Delores' struggle. I look back to the day I surrendered my way for God's way. I was standing in a restaurant parking lot when I said to God, "I don't care any longer what I look like, I don't care what I eat. I just want to make peace with food. Most of all, I want peace with you, Lord. I will now do whatever you tell me to do." I chose His peace over my own desire for thinness. I chose his new way over my old way. I chose unfamiliar territory over the familiar.

Right before my decision to release everything to God, I was in a whirlwind of familiar options that I had depended on before, "There must be a diet that has all the answers," I'd think to myself. "Maybe I'm addicted to sugar! Maybe I just need to cut out all bread, all carbohydrates. Yes, that's it! I have a chemical dependency and once I start eating processed food, I cannot stop! ... No, I know what I will do ... cut out all dinners at night. I will eat only breakfast and lunch and a snack ... a late snack or ... maybe one of those diet shakes ... What if I just run longer or do sit-ups every day, a hundred sit-ups, twice a day, and drink lots of water, lots and lots of water. Yes, that's it, I will drown myself in water and that will curb my appetite and help me lose weight ... I could always take some pills, some diet pills that keep me from getting hungry ..."

Do any of these options sound familiar to you? Do you relate to the desperateness of my cry? When I finally gave up the fight as I knew it and just asked God what to do, a miracle began. I invited the Lord into my kitchen, into my eating habits, my exercise and my health in general. Once I quietly surrendered, I found myself in a place of peace. I didn't need to lose the weight before the peace came. I was instantly at peace and I actually started to love myself as I was, even before there were evident changes in my behavior and my body.

It all happened when I admitted that I did not have the answers and I needed supernatural help. When we come to the end of ourselves, we are ready to spill ourselves out to God, and only then is He given license to respond to our call.

Right there in that parking lot, the Lord gave me my first instructions for His way. He told me to eat breakfast. Those two words meant more than just eating a piece of toast and an egg in the morning. They represented a relinquishing of control and that was scary. He was asking me to quit starving myself in the morning to compensate for nightly binges. I was to eat like a normal person, end the cycle of dieting, and trust Him with the next step. Leaning hard upon Him, the next morning, I did it. I ate breakfast and waited for God to come through.

Faithful as always, God came through. He started teaching me how to live each day, how to eat, exercise, rest and even how to think of myself. The battle to re-assume the controls was not yet finished though and I still have to be on the watch for alternative plans that entice me with their quick-fix solutions. As each diet idea or extreme pattern of living enter my mind, I reject them and let God come through. Now instead of noisily seeking out answers, I quietly listen. I listen for God to tell me what to do.

I was once told that Jesus can dare to claim your life because He knows that He is the only one that can control you without destroying you. All other ways of life which seek to control your appetite, your moods, your contentment and your success, will eventually bring death. Jesus is the only one that we can get extreme about without forfeiting life. Every other area has its place in a balance that only God can orchestrate.

When it comes to food and exercise, God's way is all about stability. We are not meant to constantly suffer intense lows and highs brought on by changing behaviors in drastic measure. We are created instead to soar like eagles upon the drafts of the wind, moving smoothly and effortlessly, with small changes and fluctuations.

---

[1] Ephesians 6:12.

[2] D. Engell. "Interdependency of food and water intake in humans." *Appetite* 10 (1988): 133-141.

[3] H.L. Jacobs. "The interaction of hunger and thirst: experimental separation of osmotic and oral-gastric factors in regulating caloric intake." *Thirst* (1964): 117-134.

[4] Julia Cameron. *The Artist's Way, the spiritual path to higher creativity* (New York, NY: Jeremy P. Tarcher/ Putnam, 1992), 29-30.

· Chapter 7 ·

Reclaiming Feared Foods

Studies have shown that restrictive dieting helps one maintain habitual binge eating. When people who have suffered from binge eating impose a strict diet upon themselves, rules at some point will be broken and the consequential feelings often include self-blame, criticism, shame, fear, sadness, guilt and depression.

There are no moral consequences behind food itself. Paul explains in 1 Corinthians, chapter 6 that "All things are lawful for me, but not all things are profitable. All things are lawful for me, but I will not be mastered by anything." (NAS)

The question is not whether a certain type of food is morally good or bad, but whether it becomes a person's master. If I eat sweet foods every time I'm upset and I can't seem to break this habit, then I am being "mastered." This "addiction mindset" can put us in a place of danger, and as Christians we are free to choose lives without addictive dependence upon anything.

If I say I'm addicted to sugar and I believe it in my heart, then I'm giving power to sugar. How can I be a conqueror over all things of the flesh when sugar has control over me and instead of one serving of ice cream, I eat half a gallon? If I believe I will consume half a bag of chips once I crunch into the first chip, then I have given power to potato chips before I even buy the bag.

When I was growing up, my mother didn't buy sweetened cereal for breakfast. We ate whole grain, low sugar cereals every morning. Once in awhile she would buy a sugary brand of cereal and my brother, sister and I would 'inhale' the whole box in a day or two. I ate that sugary cereal so fast the milk could barely soften the thick, sugary wafers, which tore the skin from the roof of my mouth as I ate.

As I grew up and started living on my own, I continued this feast or famine pattern. The consequences moved from simply tearing the skin on the roof of my mouth to long binges and deep self-hate. It always began with a "sterile" home environment. Not a single cabinet contained chips or cookies, sugar cereals or crackers. I cleared my home of every trace of temptations. The restrictions I placed on myself at home created temptation-free eating. I ate pure, healthy food every day.

Then someone would invite me to a party, or a dinner with friends, or the office would celebrate an employee's birthday. Every time I was in an environment that offered "forbidden foods," I went crazy. I would eat the first serving, swearing to myself that I would not eat another bite. But then the second and third servings always followed. Sometimes I would help "clean-up" after dinner at a friend's house and find myself secretly eating off people's plates in the kitchen!

When I got home, I would eat whatever concoction I could create to add to my binge. "May as well," I'd think. "Because you're gonna pay tomorrow – NO MORE sugar or refined flour for you! You better enjoy food while you can." I would honestly make the commitment to myself that I would never eat that "bad food" again.

The next day I would command adherence to pure eating as if I were part of a fruit and veggie Gestapo. All would be well in my world – until the next invitation to a social gathering where forbidden food was available.

There is a Biblical principle at work in this kind of thinking. When I live by the dictates of man, "do not taste, do not handle," I'm living by the law and not by grace. Paul says that these practices have the appearance of wisdom but are of no value against the indulgences of the flesh. Paul talks about dying with Christ from the basic principles of the world. If I am following this precept, then why am I fasting from white sugar, white flour, and all food after nine at night, expecting these practices to tilt the war for my soul in favor of my spirit over my flesh?[2]

The futility of living by the dictates of man actually **increases** our struggle with food. When a certain type of food is placed "off limits," it becomes more desirable. Therefore, legalizing "forbidden foods" is an effective way of breaking the all-or-nothing mindset of restrictive dieting.

BINGE RATING EXERCISE

Categorizing "feared foods" along a more flexible continuum and then slowly re-introducing them into regular eating is a successful method explained by Joyce D. Nash, Ph.D. in her book, *Binge No More.*[3] If you don't apply anything else in this book to your life, try to grasp this concept ... it will jumpstart your healing. It will challenge the diet mindset and show you a better way of thinking about food.

She suggests making a list of all the foods you're constantly banning from your life, only to binge on them later. Rate them according to how much you "fear" them. Give a "High-Fear" rating to the most feared, a "Low-Fear" rating to the least feared, and a "Medium-Fear" rating to foods in between. Try not to give the same ranking to all of your forbidden foods. Then reintroduce them into your planned meals or snacks a little at a time. Begin with the "Low-Fear" foods and after successfully eating them in normal portions and at normal times, move to the "Medium-Fear" and then to the "High-Fear" foods.

Try to include one or two of these feared foods with your meals each week. Be sure to do so when you are not overly stressed or overly hungry. The idea is to prove to yourself that you can eat a feared food in moderation and not have it automatically trigger a binge or cause you to gain weight. Also remember that you can always eat that food again on another day, and therefore, it is not necessary to go overboard now.

When I started this process, I found I couldn't have ice cream in the house. I would consume a gallon in a few days. It was a "High-Fear" food. So I chose to avoid it for awhile. Then I tried an item on my "Low-Fear" list – cookies individually wrapped in plastic packaging. I ate one at snack-time between lunch and dinner. That worked well because I wasn't crazy about them. Cookies were not in any way connected to my past. I can remember my mother making cookies at Christmas but that was all. They didn't represent mom or home or love in any way. So this was a good food to begin with – little emotional connection, yet certainly not considered a healthy food option for weight loss. I feared cookies but I wasn't obsessed with them.

The separate wrapping also helped me limit my consumption to one portion. An entire container of forbidden food was too enticing for a binge. I later applied this same practice to ice cream and bought individually wrapped ice cream sandwiches, cones and bars. In fact, I would encourage you to use only foods that come individually wrapped as you start this exercise. Move to bags and boxes only after you have experienced continued success with the portions in serving-size packaging.

The freedom I experienced in eating cookies once a day was a major miracle for me. It was amazing to realize I wasn't physically addicted to sugar. I had spent most of my life thinking I had a chemical addiction to sweets. I believed if I ate one portion of sugar, I would lose control and eat until I was stuffed. Now that I had rebuffed this myth, for the first time in twenty years, I felt free to eat what I wanted.

More importantly, as I ate cookies as part of my regular diet, they lost their attractiveness. Eating them when I wasn't emotionally upset broke the familiar chain of events (emotionally upset = sugar). Now that I ate sugar as a regular part of my day I didn't want it as much when I was upset. The "association power" within the cookies was decreasing.

By routinely eating food that had normally been prohibited, the excitement diminished. Over time I was left with feelings of disinterest in the once-desired food. I started to almost disdain my mid-afternoon snack. When this happened, I would introduce something else on my "Low-Fear" list. Eventually my "Medium-Fear" food list became "Low-Fear" so I would practice eating those foods. When I finished with that list, I moved to my "High-Fear" list (which was now in a "Low-Fear" category) and today I can have a couple gallons of ice cream in my freezer without them inviting a problem. Miracle of miracles!

Disordered eating is also strongly associated with restricted self-nurturance. The sweets I allowed myself to eat each day became a form of self-nurturance that was unfamiliar at first, but enjoyable as I got used to it. [4]

Another observation made when re-introducing "Forbidden Foods" into my life was the cost of the food. I find that if I buy cheap, junk food like potato chips or caramel corn, I actually feel like "cheap junk" and I am more likely to binge on it. If instead I buy healthy, somewhat expensive food like wheat-free, organic chocolate chip cookies, I feel more valued and I almost never binge on this kind of food.

By keeping my house well stocked with enjoyable food, a third observation came to light. When I practiced my old methods of weight loss, I used to allow my cupboards and refrigerator to go bare. It was just another self-deprivation technique. An old tape was playing, "You're not worth having all the food you need and want." But with "Low-Fear" foods in the cupboards, this old tape in my head was being destroyed. It takes work to keep groceries in the house and even more effort to plan healthy meals that take time to prepare. Yet these very practices will encourage self-caring and lasting change.

FAULTY THEORIES FOR DECREASING BINGE EATING

"Eating when you are hungry and stopping when you are full" is misinformed and unhelpful advice to those who struggle with abnormal eating habits. The normal mechanisms that control hunger and fullness are no longer understood by someone who has been eating irregularly. One must relearn how to identify these signals and make eating choices accordingly, but this will occur only after some time of eating normally.

Avoiding all white flour and white sugar is a popular, extreme method of restriction. The theory of carbohydrate craving has been claimed as a reason for the maintenance of abnormal eating. The idea is that the body is addicted to certain processed carbohydrates and upon consuming one portion, the body gives off signals not unlike those experienced by an alcoholic upon taking the first drink. These signals are so intense that the second, third and fourth portions cannot be denied and the person is sent off on a binge. The solution for this person is to avoid these foods completely.

This theory, however, is not scientifically supported in research.

In my personal experience, I have found that the emotional addiction or as I explained it in chapter five, the Antecedent/Behavior Association, is far more powerful than any physical addiction. Connected to Alcoholics Anonymous is a support group called Overeaters Anonymous (OA) that uses the Twelve Step process of recovery in helping people break their unhealthy relationship with food. There are many people committed to OA who live according to the doctrine of physical addiction to white flour and sugar. While in my twenties, I attended OA for several years and applied their program to my eating by avoiding all foods that included sugar or flour within the first three ingredients listed on the back of any package of food.

I didn't find lasting results with OA. The lasting changes I came to understand were instead based upon a healing God gave me in regard to the reasons why I went to food for help and comfort. I go into deeper detail on this topic in a later chapter. For now, I want to simply challenge this addiction theory. I no longer believe I am addicted to white flour and sugar and I eat both in moderation. Even in cases where physical addiction to a certain drug is evident, most ex-addicts will admit that the emotional withdrawal is always the greater foe compared to the physical withdrawal.

NORMAL EATING

The following list was taken from *Binge No More* by Joyce D. Nash, PH.D. and I found it an excellent guide to follow.

a. Eating three meals and one to two planned snacks daily at regular, consistent times of the day, regardless of hunger.

b. Allowing no more than 3-4 hours between eating episodes

c. Initially, focus on when, not what you eat.

d. Don't skip meals

e. Eat only planned snacks

f. Get back on track as soon as possible if you slip

g. After you are comfortable eating at pre-established times, begin to introduce healthier food choices.

h. Avoid dieting that involves restrictive eating, restricting calories, or restricting specific foods or macronutrients

i. Reintroduce "forbidden foods" into meal plan following Binge Rating Exercise

COUNTING CALORIES AND SLOW CHANGE

Let's go back to that piece of chocolate birthday cake and dollop of ice cream at my friend's house in the previous chapter. Why wouldn't 600 calories be a problem for a person trying to lose weight? The answer is in the perception we have about food and calories and change.

I will illustrate. A sedentary woman has been living with forty extra pounds since her last pregnancy two years ago. Her weight has stabilized but she is ready to lose that forty extra pounds. In order for this woman to lose one pound of fat in a week, she must eat 3,500 calories less than what she normally does. She would need to cut down her caloric intake by 500 calories per day to lose a pound in a week. Most people do not have a concept of how many calories 500 calories represents.

Most overweight people eat between 2,000 and 3,000 calories each day. Therefore, 500 calories represent 1/4 to 1/6 of this woman's calories every day just to lose one pound. Now of course she could exercise 250 calories off and just cut back 250 calories in her diet to meet the 500-calorie goal. This would be more realistic and certainly more balanced in approach.

The point is that losing one pound of fat in one week is not easy. It takes commitment and consistency. The flip side to this is that once a person loses a pound of fat in a week, it would take just as much commitment of eating and not exercising to gain that 3,500 calories back.

So a piece of chocolate birthday cake with ice cream is not going to ruin a person's diet, it will simply slow down the progress. The cake and ice cream may not be such a bad idea, especially if it is a "Low-Fear" food for you – just make sure it is one portion. The truth is, one portion of cake and ice cream will probably stop a binge from occurring and the amount of calories ingested in a binge is usually double to triple 600 calories.

As we have discovered, God usually authors change in our lives with consistent, small steps, not cavernous leaps and bounds.

Releasing our extreme thinking for God's method of change will bring about the success we were created to taste without the hills and valleys of dramatic living and all the painful consequences connected. Are you convinced of this?

If you're not convinced of this concept of eating normally and still losing weight, ask yourself one question. If you ate normal meals every day, never indulging in a second portion, never eating out of emotion, and if you exercised moderately four times each week, would you lose weight in a year? The answer will inevitably be yes. Keep this in mind as you continue to read. In the next chapter we will look at some scriptures that support this slower, deeper process.

---

[1] E. Stice, C. Ziemba, J. Margolis, and P. Flick. "The dual pathway model differentiates bulimics, subclinical bulimics, and controls: Testing the continuity hypothesis" *Behavior Therapy* 27 (1996): 531-549.

[2] Colossians 2: 11-23.

[3] Joyce D. Nash. *Binge No More, Your Guide to Overcoming Disordered Eating* (Oakland, CA:New Harbinger Publications, 1999), 132-137.

[4] A.K. Lehman and J. Rodin. "Styles of self-nurturance and disordered eating" *Journal of consulting and Clinical Psychology* 57 (1989): 117-122.

Chapter 8

Slow & Steady Wins the Race

We have looked at how important it is to release our diet mindset for God's mindset in order to move into lifestyle change. God's written word is full of examples of this truth.

Before the children of Israel entered into Canaan, the Promised Land, God made it clear He didn't plan to give them complete rule of the land all at once. He gave it to them bit by bit, territory by territory.

> Deuteronomy 7:22, *"And the LORD your God will drive out those nations before you little by little; you will be unable to destroy them at once, lest the beasts of the field become too numerous for you."*

The nations driven out by the Lord represent the enemies of our lives that must be destroyed in order for us to reign in our "promised land" of a healthy spirit, soul and body. These enemy nations include behaviors such as binge eating and sedentary living. They also include the results of these behaviors such as hypertension, heart disease, and diabetes. God destroys these enemies gradually, slowly. He applies His power this way for a good reason. Anyone can succeed in attaining initial possession of the "promised land." But there is another enemy to consider, and this sort of enemy can stop us from making permanent habitation.

These enemies are the beasts of the field. They offer a different challenge, for they are deeply ingrained in the territory. They are the values, attitudes and beliefs that are within our territory, and they take longer to change. Like animals that have come to know a particular habitat for generations; they are profoundly set in our minds and hearts, regulating our decisions and habitual patterns.

Many people can lose weight for a season, begin a walking routine outside when the weather is nice or quit drinking soda for Lent. But how do these same people make it a lifestyle change? By permanent habitation. The beasts of the field must be addressed. So God, in His sovereignty, moves us in gradually.

> As Matthew Henry explains,
> *"Note, the wisdom of God is to be observed in the gradual advances of the church's interests. It is in real kindness to the church that its enemies are subdued by little and little; for thus we are kept upon our guard, and in a continual dependence upon God. Corruptions are thus driven out of the hearts of God's people; not all at once, but by little and little; the old man is crucified, and therefore dies slowly. God, in his providence, often delays mercies, because we are not ready for them. Canaan has room enough to receive Israel, but Israel is not numerous enough to occupy Canaan."*[1]

An alcoholic can be healed of the physical dependency upon alcohol, but it is the paradigm of self that must also change in order for the physical manifestation to remain. A person dependent upon food as a source of comfort can begin to exercise and eat healthier, but again the understanding they have of who they are in relation to food must also adjust when seeking lasting change. I don't believe lifetime change comes through physical manifestations or spiritual healing. The answer is found in both. The Lord moves out the nations **while** the beasts of the field dwindle in strength. The important point is that it is not usually accomplished with great speed.

With our heart-felt, desperate cry for change, God conquers "a nation of enemies." If you're struggling with binge eating and you have come to a place where you're willing to submit to His method of weight loss, He is then in the position to conquer one of your "nations." He may introduce you to a potential exercise buddy. He may give you the motivation to start drinking water instead of soda. Just be mindful, the work will be slow.

Let's review the principle,

Spirit, soul and body are connected and affect one another.

The process of change stated in chapter four includes the battle between the flesh and the spirit. When our spirits are in control of our souls and our souls then direct the behaviors of our bodies, we can experience an increase in health. If I expect my body to change, my soul must first change. And soul change is long, hard work. Jack Hayford explains this phenomenon in his book, *Rebuilding the Real You.*[2]

He uses the story of Nehemiah and the rebuilding of the walls of Jerusalem to parallel the work of the Holy Spirit upon our souls. At the beginning of the story, we discover that the people of the city had rebuilt the temple 70 years prior, but the walls were still in complete ruin. Hayford explains that the temple, which had been rebuilt comparatively fast, represents our spirits when we are born again. Just as we confess Jesus as Lord and Savior, we are at that instant, born again. The wall and its gates, however, represent our souls and when we enter into this new relationship with Jesus, the soul is placed into a process where continual renewal is needed every day. This is the part of us that relegates the physical health of the body.

Nehemiah was a leader of the Jews and at the time, working for the Persian emperor, Artaxerxes, as his consultant. Upon hearing that the walls of Jerusalem were still in ruins, he requested time off from his job to begin the task of rebuilding the wall. He didn't ask for two weeks paid vacation. He knew that even a year off would not suffice. He instead asked for twelve years! Nehemiah did this because he understood the work he set out to accomplish would demand incremental steps and a great deal of time. Just as Nehemiah set out to lead the task of rebuilding the wall, in the same way the Holy Spirit sets out to change our souls – our mind, will, and emotions. This also takes a great amount of time and small steps.

Are you ready to release your methods of change for God's method? Are you willing to give up your agenda, timetable, and perception of yourself in order to embrace God's plan for your health? Until you are, you will never experience lasting change. Pray for this humility to come. God will faithfully remind you that He has the better plan, even if it does involve small steps and slow progress.

We serve a conditional God. We take that first step and then He follows with great reward. Once you make the decision to obey His way, we will then be able to move into the next chapters of change. If you are ready, pray the following prayer aloud,

Dear Heavenly Father, in the name of Jesus Christ, I confess that I have tried losing weight and mastering food my own way. I am tired of my own way. It doesn't work. I want Your way.

I ask forgiveness from You for:

(include any of the following that are applicable to you)

1. Disobedience to Your voice regarding dieting
2. Impatience and self-hate toward myself in regard to my body and my eating
3. Addiction to the highs and lows of the diet cycle
4. Fear of the truths underlying my overeating

I release all of my diets, appetite suppressants, quick fix plans and extreme exercise programs to You. I choose to hear Your voice regarding my relationship with food. I repent, Lord. I choose Your method for change in the name of Jesus Christ. Thank You for Your love. I receive healing from Your Holy Spirit.

"For my thoughts are not your thoughts, Nor are your ways My ways,' says the Lord. 'For as the heavens are higher than the earth, so are My ways higher than your ways, and My thoughts than your thoughts."[3]

[1] Matthew Henry. *Matthew Henry's Commentary on the Bible* (Peabody, MA: Hendrickson Publishers, 1997), Exodus 23:20.

[2] Jack W. Hayford. *Rebuilding the Real You* (Ventura, CA: Regal Books, 1986), 26.

[3] Isaiah 55:8-9.

Chapter 9

Let's Be Honest

STEP 1: Release our methods of change for God's method
STEP 2: Examine a negative behavior — FRUIT

What do you see when you look at yourself in a full-length mirror? Have you done it recently? Have you done it with all the lights on, stark naked, front view, side view, rear view? O.K., so you may not be open to doing this, so how do you feel just thinking about it? Filled with shame? Sadness? Anger?

Can I tell you something shocking? God looks at you in a full-length mirror every moment of every day. He sees all of you. He knows you better than you know yourself. What does He see in that mirror? He sees Himself. He sees God incarnate staring back. This is not a lie. He is not sugar-coating the reality of your image. He sees your fat, your rolls, your scars and dimples. He knows all about your stretch marks and how you got them, and every place your eyes roam, He has already discovered. He is not pretending. He is not forgetting. He takes it all in and He loves you. Because of Jesus, the Father God truly loves you just as you are.[1,2]

Until you see yourself in a full-length mirror – assessing both your weaknesses and strengths, and at the same time, knowing that God is in that mirror, you will not move one step closer to the balance He has called you to. We must face the reality of our lives – look at the consequences of our behavior in a stark light and take in God's love for us in response to this reality.

Alcoholics Anonymous uses this same powerful tool of observation in their 12-step process. Step Four is "Make a searching and fearless moral inventory of ourselves," step number Eight is "Make a list of all persons we had harmed ..." and "Continued to take personal inventory ... "[3] is step number ten. These steps bring the reality of excessive drinking and its consequences into full view. Only then can a person struggling with alcohol make and keep the changes necessary for a lifetime of sobriety.

EXAMINE

TAKING INVENTORY

Sometimes I have trouble realizing what it meant when Jesus died on the cross for me. The bizarre truth of one man's death wiping out all of my sin is difficult to grasp in an intellectual way. One way of bringing that truth home is through this type of thorough inventory. Taking a picture of myself in a bathing suit helps me see myself for what I am and the consequences of my sin. Then I can turn to God for forgiveness and help. It's in seeing ourselves completely that we can stand in amazement of God's continued love for us.

Now let's consider the essential step of accurate observation and how it can serve as a form of confession. As you make accurate observations about your behavior, then share these observations with God and others, you can move toward permanent change.

> *"If we say that we have no sin, we deceive ourselves, and the truth is not in us. If we confess our sins, He is faithful and just to forgive us our sins and to cleanse us from all unrighteousness."*[1]

CONFESSION — WHAT IS IT?

The idea of confession may conjure up discomfort and feelings of guilt. Not surprising. We are all afraid someone will discover we're weak and limited in strength and control, and perhaps we won't be loved or respected.

In my journey to health, I have come to embrace confession and see it as a gift. It's like the tug that pulls the sliver out of your finger, it hurts for the moment but the relief it brings always supersedes the prior pain. Confession will take you into greater levels of health in spirit, soul and body.

When clients first meet with me, I take all kinds of measurements to gauge their health. I measure blood pressure, waist size, weight, muscle strength, heart strength and even flexibility. Together we then compare these results with other people in the same age and gender. I have witnessed the grief of men and women whose results register in the "poor" category. The silence following a weigh-in that hasn't occurred in years is all too telling. As I measure their waist, bust and hips, I have seen tears stream down my clients' faces. There is, in all of us, sorrow over the consequences of negative behavior. And yet that pain is a gift.

While taking these measurements, I listen to them grieve, but I refuse to downplay the reality of their state. It's part of the process necessary for change. At the same time, I make sure to encourage each client and remind them of God's love and how we can now begin a healing process with God in regard to our eating.

There are several forms of accurate observation. These observations will ultimately lead to confession. Written observation, counseling and clothing size are a few. By reading the differing methods of accurate observation and how they can serve you in your journey, I hope you too will learn to see confession as friend – not foe.

WRITTEN OBSERVATION

I used to feel like my life was one long binge. I was never aware of the specific times of day and days of the week I chose to binge. I thought I just ate a lot. Then during one of my classes on behavior change, I learned that examining a negative behavior pattern was essential to altering that behavior. So I began logging my binges. Although I had little hope this would help me, I was desperate, so I tried it anyway.

I hated listing all the food I was eating during my binges – seeing it on paper caused too much shame. Yet I didn't mind writing out the specific days and times when I binged. I used a monthly calendar and wrote, "binge" on the days I overate, including the time of day. After a few weeks, a surprising pattern emerged. There were the occasional binges during the week, but without fail, every Sunday night was my all-time worst period for bingeing.

I scrutinized this time period. What was so significant about Sunday night? What happens every Sunday that could cause this eruption in negative behavior? And why Sunday night, and not Sunday morning or afternoon? I discovered the reasons for these specific binges as I applied steps three and four to my life, which we will cover in detail later.

Prior to this revelation, I was convinced that I ate endlessly without rhyme or reason. Once I became honest with myself and examined my negative behavior through written observation, something I once saw as erratic was actually predictable. Now I was closer to understanding my behavior and I could get help to alter it.

Let's consider, in greater detail, why written observation is so important.

Food logs, journals and observation charts help us look at our behavior with objectivity. **While memory loss and emotional distortion of the facts** can limit our success at changing behavior, examination through written observation can decrease these natural tendencies.

MEMORY LOSS

As humans, we don't remember the past accurately. Recording the facts, (i.e. calories in each day), allows us to recall what really happened and enables us to make wise decisions based upon these facts.

A recent study involved a group of people who had continually failed at losing weight. Researchers asked them to write down everything they had eaten that past week. During the following week the researchers then asked the participants to eat only the food they had written down. The group did this the next week and when they were weighed, all of them lost weight. This supports the notion that we're often not taking notice of what we're eating and our recall of past behavior is inaccurate because of memory loss.

EMOTIONAL DISTORTION OF THE FACTS

All through my teens, twenties, and early thirties I lived according to the swings of my emotions. Regardless of outward appearances, if I was experiencing a time of emotional upheaval, I felt like the size of a behemoth. I constantly practiced extreme diets and exercise and my weight fluctuated radically through a twenty-pound range.

Once I started logging my behavior in my mid-thirties, I began applying basic scientific facts of nutrition to my life ... without my emotions relegating my lifestyle. My new, targeted behavior was simple – no more bingeing, dieting or extreme exercise. I ate three meals and one snack every day and exercised without excess (eating plan details were covered in Chapter 7). It was hard to believe that this kind of behavior would not produce a bigger body. Yet as I started eating and exercising at normal levels, my weight did not increase. In fact, I actually lost weight. I could never have stayed consistent with this new, moderate method of eating and exercising if I had not depended upon the facts of written observation to help fight my old, extreme mindset.

I kept a daily food log, weighed and measured myself each week and monitored my exercise on a calendar. I had to resist the fear that said I was going to get fat by living a "normal" life. But the evidence was clear: these observable facts of pounds lost and inches decreasing helped me persist. I only practiced logging information for the first six months and then I started to wean off strict record keeping.

Five years into my healing, I still practice logging. I continue to weigh myself on a scale each week and when I experience a fear of weight gain, I measure my chest, waist, hips and thighs to further support the scale's numbers. These facts counter my fears and have a way of setting me free. Here is a biblical principle in action,

Confession is good for the soul – accurate records shed light on darkness and separate fact from fiction.

As you consider your behavior of overeating, negative emotions will surely surface. There is nothing wrong with emotions in and of themselves, but they can cause us to lose objectivity. Though they help reveal hidden pain, they often paint a picture that is not factual. The more accurate and thorough the recorded data, the clearer the delineation between feelings and behaviors. Emotions do not have to dictate our behaviors but, *without knowing the difference between feelings and behaviors, we are enslaved to a process we don't understand.*

Upon beginning their journey toward health, many of my clients find that they obsess over the numbers they must record.

Counting calories, measuring food and weighing oneself on a scale can mistakenly become the focal point of a person's life. This is not the purpose of God's plan to health. There are plenty of diets that do this and we know they don't offer a lifestyle change. However, obsessing over numbers is normal, yet short-lived if a person is balancing this method of record keeping with the excavation of the reasons behind unhealthy behavior (revealed in steps three and four).

CONSISTENCY IS KEY

Carol was a client of mine who needed to lose a great deal of weight. She had become obese through extreme binge eating and starvation. While working on her program, Carol became pregnant. She continued meeting with me in order to keep her nutritional intake at an optimal level and her calorie amount normal so she would not gain too much weight during pregnancy. Many years prior, when she gave birth to her first daughter, she had gained over 95 pounds. She didn't want to gain that much weight again. She remembered how difficult it was for her to breathe and move in the last three months of that pregnancy and this caused great fear to arise. This fear then fueled her desire to hide the facts from herself and me by avoiding weighing in or writing down her food intake. She missed appointments for several weeks.

After a while, we met. She weighed in and found that she had gained four pounds. She panicked and became bound in fear regarding her ability to achieve her objective. I doubted she had gained the four pounds over a few days, but instead felt it was due to a relapse that had lasted for several weeks. If she had been diligent in her record keeping and honest with herself during the full program cycle, we could have prevented this sudden surprise and the destructive consequences that followed. Unfortunately she quit working with me and I haven't heard from her since.

I often work with clients who openly share their eating and exercise habits thoroughly until they hit a wall or lose control. The shame we feel in being honest about our negative behavior during a relapse causes us to recoil and "sweep under the rug" everything we're doing wrong. However, it is exactly at these times where we must be diligent in approaching our negative behavior with thorough honesty, believing that God comes to our rescue in our weakness.

We need to see unhealthy behavior as a helpful marker calling out a warning, "DANGER! EXPLOSIVES BURIED HERE!" Unhealthy behavior warns us of a place in our hearts that needs our attention. If we ignore a heart issue or refute it, we lose an opportunity to walk in greater freedom in an area that tends to ensnare us and block us from a more intimate love relationship with the Lover of our soul.

You may be wondering, "Do I have to count my calories for the rest of my life?" At the beginning of your journey you must be vigilant in detailed record keeping. In time, as you uncover the roots of your behavior, you can eventually wean off the daily calorie counting. The numbers served you well in understanding yourself, and you can let them go, trusting that you will continue to see change because of the new revelations they provided.

Yet even long after a person finds success in changing a behavior, record keeping can still be useful. Old habits have a way of coming back. After several years of healthy, normal eating, I still have slips and find myself bingeing on food I do not need. By simply writing out my food intake for a couple days, I can start the process that gets me back on track again.

When a distorted view of the truth has held us hostage for a long season in the past, we can often still live there even when the present is different. Accurate measurements and written observations break this distortion.

COUNSELING

Another method of accurate observation that serves as confession is counseling. Meeting with qualified professional counselors can help us uncover unhealthy behaviors and tendencies quickly and efficiently. The neutrality of the counselor is helpful, and I'm always amazed by the positive

EXAMINE

results of only a few sessions with a counselor. Counselors invite us to listen to ourselves. They have the training and ability to separate emotions from facts so that problems become clearer and solutions easier to find.

Psychotherapists, pastors and even good friends who know how to listen can counsel us effectively. Yet it is important to remember that the Holy Spirit is the Counselor God sent us. We need to attribute any truth revealed to us in counseling as the work of the Holy Spirit in our lives. He works through all kinds of instruments of grace.

What qualities should you look for in a good counselor? One characteristic essential for healthy accountability is love. People that know and love themselves have the necessary self-esteem to assist you in reaching your personal health goals. Out of this place of self-caring, a counselor will exude the essential trait of honesty. One must be dedicated enough to your growth to tell you the truth, even when it hurts.

Experience is another important quality to look for in a counselor. If the person you meet with has "walked in your shoes," then they are more likely to empathize and relate effectively to your situation. Training is also a plus but sometimes life's experiences alone can allow a person to hold you firm to your commitments without formal schooling.

Spiritual agreement is of utmost importance. As a Christian, you cannot receive complete healing from a person that does not possess the same basic beliefs that you hold. Worse yet, you can be directed into unbiblical paths that deny the existence of God. I know many Christians that guard against counseling of any sort because of bad experiences that led them into self-healing instead of biblical healing based on the gospel of Jesus Christ.

Choosing a counselor with the guidance of the Holy Spirit, is therefore paramount and when working with a Christian counselor, it should be clearly emphasized that the Holy Spirit is a participant in each meeting, leading and guiding both counselor and counselee into God's agenda for healing.

CLOTHING SIZE

As I lost weight over the years, I still had the mindset that I was my old, larger size. When I began to get smaller, I continued wearing the same size clothes. I was comfortable wearing baggy pants and tops, dark colors and solids. Well meaning friends and family would encourage me to wear clothes that complimented my body instead of hiding it behind dark, draping fabrics. I met these suggestions with disdain.

I couldn't imagine revealing the body I had hated for years. Yet as God changed my heart and I began seeing my worth through His eyes, I started to feel comfortable in better fitting clothes. It was a struggle at first. Watching the size of my waist and hips decrease encouraged me to identify with the new person God was carving out for me as I changed.

Now I wear fitted shorts, patterned, sleeveless tops and even the often-avoided white pants. The sizes in my wardrobe have dropped four times during my healing and yet I am still amazed that I can fit these smaller sizes. Sometimes I think to myself, "If I pull the right lever, I will expand to my true, heavy size once again." To combat this emotional distortion, I used to apply the exercise of opening closet doors and reading each tag on my pants and skirts until I was satisfied that these new sizes were really the same clothes that fit my body. The reality of those tag numbers spoke to this distortion and again, I was set free from the lie I once believed.

As we lose weight God's way, our clothing is a form of examination. It is important to tailor suits and pants to fit us and to buy updated styles in sizes that truly fit. Tucking in shirts, wearing belts and putting on light colors may all be part of the celebration for the new person you are becoming!

All three of these methods of examination – written observation, counseling and clothing size are powerful. We can use them together in the process of change.

The principle of examining a negative behavior pattern is used in many parts of our lives. I have a friend who consults with people on how to conduct their finances. He requires his clients to account for every penny spent. A person cannot assess how change is to take place if he is not aware of his present financial state and a consultant cannot help without these detailed facts at his perusal. Sports performance is improved with the use of video reviews and systematic breakdowns of an athlete's technique.

Written observation is routine in the business world, education, and the medical environment. Yet, when it comes to personal behavior, we often blow a whistle and yell, "Stop! You can mess with me at work and in school, but as for my personal life, I get a break!" Yet, we know as Christians this is misguided thinking. The Word of God says that we are to give our entire lives over to the guidance of the Holy Spirit, without exception. We simply need to be accountable in every area of life to activate our liberty in Christ Jesus.

---

[1] 1 John 1:8-10.

[2] 1 John 4:18-19.

[3] "Is there an Alcoholic in Your Life?" (Alcoholics Anonymous World Services, Inc., 1976).

Chapter 10

Here is Your Miracle!

STEP 1: Release our methods of change for God's method
STEP 2: Examine a negative behavior — FRUIT
STEP 3: Express our feelings to God about our behavior and listen to His response — MOVE TO ROOTS

With a tear-stained face, Renee launched into prayer asking God for forgiveness.

"O Heavenly Father above, I ask you to please forgive me for not trusting You with my job. Help me love these people that have hurt me."

While her prayer seemed sincere, I knew she was not being completely open and honest with God.

Renee had arrived at our appointment with her head held down in shame. She had again resumed her old habit of overeating at night and hadn't exercised all week. After we sought the reasons behind her setback, she shared with me that she had been spending more time at the office than usual. As a result, she was tired. She was also angry. Some clients were suing her employer and she was very upset with them. They were about to destroy her employer's welfare and thereby her own job security.

Unexpressed fear was the deep, underlying foe that supported all her feelings and subsequent negative behavior (overworking, overeating, and sedentary living). Every extra bite of food she took had "medicated" her fear, temporarily anesthetizing her apprehension of losing her job. Yet as we discussed her work environment, I could see the burden of this fear somewhat lifted and her countenance change as she admitted her thoughts to me. Simply by sharing with me, her feelings were validated as real and the power behind them released.

I liken this scenario to a teapot of water reaching the boiling point. Something has to take the pressure of the steam. My teapot spout whistles so loud that I can hear it on the other side of the house. The more steam that it creates, the louder and higher the whistle becomes.

Consider the whistling spout as the negative behavior you are trying to decrease (overeating). When I am upset, I turn to food and eat with great ferocity. The greater the emotion, the more I eat. I am "whistling" in my own way.

If I release steam somehow, there is no need for the whistle. Likewise, if I express my emotions and "let off steam," the need to overeat vanishes, just like the whistle that falls silent when I take the top off the teapot.

How do we apply this phenomenon to overeating? The answer lies in ***Step 3, Express our feelings about our behavior to God…***

Back to Renee. She had exposed her emotions to me, but I then asked her to pray to God and share the same with Him. (I practice this transfer as often as possible for He is the Almighty Counselor, far more able and always available).

However, in her prayer, Renee didn't voice the same concerns she had shared with me just a moment prior. Instead, she moved into a place of familiar, religious jargon. She prayed a prayer of "oughts" instead of her true, heartfelt thoughts.

As I held her hands, I softly prompted her to tell God what she had just told me, share her true feelings, share her heart. After a long pause, she responded, "I am angry, God. I feel like these people are hurting me but I don't know why." Her emotions choked her words and her weeping came to the surface.

"Now we are getting somewhere," I thought to myself.

She continued, "I have been so happy in this job. I know You will help me find another place of employment, but I don't want to look for another job! I want things to stay as they are … but I pray You will have Your will, whatever that is."

The gist of Renee's second prayer is much like the one Jesus prayed in the Garden of Gethsemane. Jesus went to God and prayed with great sorrow. He did not hide his emotions from His Heavenly Father. He shared His heart, His fears, and His doubts to God as a man acquainted with human grief. Matthew Henry explains it this way,

"He begs that this cup might *pass from him*, that is, that he might avoid the sufferings now at hand; or, at least, that they might be shortened. This intimates no more than that he was really and truly Man, and as a Man he could not but be averse to pain and suffering. This is the first and simple act of man's will – to start back from that which is sensibly grievous to us, and to desire the prevention and removal of it."[1]

Until we acknowledge to God and ourselves this "first and simple act of man's will," our prayers are simply dishonest before God. Honesty is crucial to effective prayer and I have found it best when we begin our prayers by openly expressing our feelings before God, just as they are, without pretense or fear.

This is the first part of Step 3 in our journey to healing – ***Express our feelings about our behavior to God*** ... How do we do this exactly? Why is it so hard?

I have found three reasons why we struggle with being honest with God in prayer. First of all, we are well practiced in religious habits. Secondly, we are more comfortable telling others of our problems than we are telling God and thirdly, we simply don't believe God cares.

EXPRESS

1. RELIGIOUS HABITS

We often try to jump over the reality of our true and present state in order to get to the part we know we **should** do. We skip the expression of our emotions and launch right into requests for forgiveness. If we were to do this with a person that was not aware of our situation, they would be very much confused. Yet we do this with God all the time. Though He knows our situations, we cannot expect to "let off steam" if we do not share our emotions with God. Honest, emotive prayer is essential for the healing of emotional eating.

In working with clients that are newly learning how to increase intimacy with God, I have found that I need to begin with basic communication skills. The majority of my clients have attended church most of their lives but have never had a deep, cathartic outpouring of prayer to God. If this sounds like you, let me offer a couple suggestions that may help.

LIMITING RELIGIOUS JARGON

As I first began sharing my feelings with God in prayer, I can remember working hard to avoid terms that I would only use in a religious setting. I purposefully thought of openings that I would use in regular conversations with good friends. I usually opened prayers with something like, "Hey there God. Thanks for being here. I'm not doing so hot right now…" These starts usually paved the way for continued honesty and a lack of false pretense and false respect.

BREAKING THE SILENCE

Praying aloud is another tool I use in prayer to increase the release of my emotions. There is something extremely cathartic about yelling aloud to the heavens. Hearing my own voice cry out for God helped me release deeper and deeper pain. In times of deep healing, my hollering prayers would transition into weeping with intermittent sobs and then weeping without words would finally submit to silence, just like a baby crying to sleep.

2. MISERY LOVES COMPANY

Another trap we often fall into is that we share our struggles with others before we share with God. I find myself calling my mother as soon as a stressful event takes place in my life. If she isn't home, I will then call friends or other family members until I at last find someone with whom I can share my grievances, beliefs and feelings. Meanwhile, between sentences, I am taking bites of unnecessary food. I often continue eating long after our conversation has ended. Why? Most people are not able to provide healing for the issues/hurts that we experience.

If we know that God is the only one who can bring about the healing we seek, why is it that we run to a friend to share our woes before offering them to God alone?

Perhaps we don't want to change. Maybe, deep down inside, we know that God will show us how we are to change, but we are more content in our misery. Maybe we would rather have someone listen and feel sorry for us. 'Misery loves company' it is true, but sadly this approach merely adds to our misery instead of allowing our hearts to be transformed to the point where God will come to our assistance. Instead of exchanging our mindsets for the mind of Christ, we muddle in our labyrinths of old thinking and wonder why we remain the same today as we were yesterday.

In holding onto these miserable habits over the years, our waist size expands, our pride becomes more implacable, and we often end up blaming God for the results.

The answer to this dilemma is in one word – humility. Pride alone stops us from going to God. Pride can kill us in the end.

3. INACCURATE PERCEPTION OF GOD

There is another possible reason for not sharing our feelings with God ... perhaps we do not trust that He cares, or that maybe He cannot love us in our sin. Yet if we know Him, apply our faith and begin to share with Him our deepest thoughts and feelings, we will find that He does care and He truly is in love with us, even in our sin.[3] During my process of healing, my perception of God has changed from a being that loves me when I do right to a Father that loves me for who I am. This change occurred as I poured out to Him and found God there, waiting for me. He was and is ever-present and inexpressively kind in His response to my cries.

Beth Moore, in her book *Praying God's Word*, explains it this way, "God never misses a single tear of the oppressed. He sees our suffering and knows the depth of our need. He anguishes yet He waits ... until the tears that have fallen on dry ground or upon the shoulders of others equally frail are poured instead before His throne. He waits – not until the oppressed cry out – but until we cry out to Him. Only then will we know the One and Only who redeems us."[2]

PRACTICAL APPLICATION

Let's go back to the prior chapter on accurate observation for a moment. As I shared in that chapter, when I started logging my binges on a monthly calendar, I realized that Sunday was the day I binged the most. It was a recurring pattern and so I examined it thoroughly. Why Sunday? In applying this third step, "Express our feelings about our behavior to God and listen to His response," I was to find out why Sunday night was so distinct. When the next Sunday came along, I put off dinnertime, instead met with God, and allowed my feelings to come to the surface.

Vividly, I remember that the feelings I felt included dread, fear and anger. As I poured out these thoughts to God, I suddenly realized that my emotions were not a response toward Sunday but instead were feelings ignited by the day around the corner. You see, Mondays always generated some serious negative emotions within me. I found myself saying, "God stop Monday from coming. I cannot face another Monday. Please don't make me go there."

At that time in my life, I was working 40 – 50 hours each week as Director of a fitness center with over 2,000 members; taught nine hours of aerobics and strength training classes and two additional exercise classes at 6:00 a.m. on Tuesdays and Thursdays in a different gym. I was also the Youth Group Leader and Praise and Worship Leader of my church, and to top it all off, I was traveling nearly 100 miles two nights each week to attend graduate school. I look at my hectic schedule now and I don't know how I survived. I was wearing myself out each week.

My only day of rest was Sunday and that wasn't really a day of rest because of my roles in the church. No wonder I dreaded Mondays. Now I understood why I binged on Sunday nights. I was trying to put off Mondays. I was placing a buffer between myself and the whipping block that waited just around the corner.

This revelation would not have occurred, though, if I had not first been honest with God about how I was feeling. This third step is essential to decreasing negative behaviors.

As I continued examining my negative behaviors of overeating with record keeping, logs and honest reflection, the honesty in my conversations with God increased. With more honesty in my conversations with God, I found that these negative behaviors never stood alone. As described in the teapot scenario, there were always coinciding feelings that went along with the sound of the "whistle." I realized that if I could get these emotions expressed to God before bingeing, I would not have reason to binge in the first place.

TIMING IS EVERYTHING

One key part to this step in decreasing bingeing is the timing. It is vital to tell God how you feel **before** the binge is over. Tell Him how you feel before you binge or tell Him how you feel while you binge just don't wait until the battle is over and you've left the kitchen to lie comatose on your favorite couch.

If you wait, you won't be in touch with your true, raw emotions. The food you eat will stifle the feelings you need to understand. When I binge, I am trying to keep my feelings inside for fear of "losing control." And yet, aren't I losing control in my eating anyway?

It is crucial to go to God AS you binge and not AFTER. This is especially difficult for people that have trouble believing that God loves them all of the time, even in the midst of committing sin. Yet, the word of God is clear on this truth, for the Father loved us before time, loves us in our sin, and loves us after our sin. Nothing can separate us from His love.[3]

EXPRESS

This was hard to do at first. When I first became cognizant of my bingeing, I then wanted to pretend that I wasn't really overeating. I would think distracting thoughts and keep my mind focused on my negative feelings. I felt like I was in a bubble as I ate. God was outside my bubble. He was, in a way, not allowed to enter, not allowed to exist during the duration of my binges.

When my binge would finally cease, and my emotions were sufficiently quelled, the guilt would start to build and eventually, God was allowed to re-surface. I would acknowledge His existence, ask for forgiveness and commit to a new way of living.

This whole charade was inevitably played out over and over again. ***Until I would allow Him to exist in my world WHILE in sin, He was not going to have an impact UPON my sin.***

The successful conversation I would have with God **during** a binge looked something like this,

God, "What's goin' on?"

Heidi, "What do you mean?"

God, "I am wondering what is happening in your heart. You seem upset."

Heidi, "Do I really? Mmmmmm ... yeah, I guess I am. Yeah, I'm upset. But I don't want to quit eating. Don't ask me to quit eating. I'm not willing to give up this food just to talk with You."

God, "That's fine. You can keep eating. Just talk to me."

Heidi, "Talk to You now? While I'm eating?"

God, "Yeah, right now. I am here. I love you."

Heidi, "How can you love me? I'm pigging out."

God, "I love you."

Heidi, "O.K., as long as You don't demand that I stop eating ... I'm ticked off."

God, "What about?"

The ensuing talk would move into my deepest hurts and pains. I would often end up crying and the food would usually fall from my hands. I did not choose to put it down, it would just lose its value, it's power. It no longer had a role to play.

When I first started having these conversations with God, and I let food drop away from my hands and my thoughts, I was astonished. It seemed too simple to be true. These moments were the biggest miracles I have ever, personally experienced. For twenty years, I had lived in bondage to this particular sin and now it was losing power over me.

I didn't have to join a convent, attend a deliverance seminar, or fast for forty days after all! I only had to believe that God loved me in my sin and that He was waiting to talk with me and take my sadness, my anger, and my disappointments into His big, loving hands.

I found more and more success sharing with God WHILE bingeing. Eventually, I began to tell God how I was feeling BEFORE bingeing. Just as an urge to binge would come to my mind, I would ponder the reasons for the urge.

I can remember sitting in my living room, telling God about my day, with an incredible desire to inhale a bunch of food. Just in talking with Him about how my day upset me, I would feel anxiety, insecurity and fear erupt from within me. Strangely enough, when I poured out to God, it felt like God was pleased even with my outpouring. Charles Spurgeon says that it is a form of worship to cry out to God in your need.

"Oh, dear heart, what is your condition? Are you torn with anguish? Are you sorely distressed? Are you lonely? Are you pushed aside? Then cry to God. No one else can help you. He is your only hope. Wonderful hope! Cry to Him, for He can help you. I tell you, in that cry of yours will be the pure and true worship that God desires. He desires a sincere cry far more than the slaughter of ten thousand rams or the pouring out of rivers of oil (Micah 6:7)... See then, poor, weeping, and distracted ones, that it is not ritualism, it is not the performance of pompous ceremonies, it is not bowing and struggling, it is not using sacred words, but it is crying to God in the hour of trouble that is the most acceptable sacrifice your spirit can bring before the throne of God."[4]

God was strong enough to listen without becoming distraught Himself, He was patient enough to not interrupt and He was wise enough to keep me from staying in my mode of introspection. I found myself believing that God cared. He cared as a loving father cares. I knew He was taking it all in. I could feel His presence. Then I would sense an amazing phenomenon – peace and a complete release from the urge to binge! I soon realized that no one else would be able to listen to me as He did. No one else understood like Him.

EXPRESS

MORE PROGRESS

"I am afraid that God will think that I am complaining and that is sin," one of my clients explained to me. Too often we have been taught that honest expression of our feelings is a form of complaint that God looks upon with contempt. This could not be further from the truth. Almost every Psalm in the Bible includes some sort of honest lament. King David pours out his complaint to God in Psalm 55 with great moaning,

> *"1 Give ear to my prayer, O God,*
> *And do not hide Yourself from my supplication.*
> *2 Attend to me, and hear me;*
> *I am restless in my complaint, and moan noisily,*

> *3 Because of the voice of the enemy,*
> *Because of the oppression of the wicked;*
> *For they bring down trouble upon me,*
> *And in wrath they hate me.*
> *4 My heart is severely pained within me,*
> *And the terrors of death have fallen upon me.*
> *5 Fearfulness and trembling have come upon me,"*

David often used this key for the healing of his heart. He knew that he needed to express, in words, what he was feeling in order for God to make changes within him. Jesus tells us in the gospels that our words are what indicate what is going on in our hearts. Our words are an expression of our hearts.[5]

After sessions of outpouring to God, I found that not all my questions were answered. I often had more questions to ask. My fears weren't turned into courage overnight and my disappointments weren't immediately forgiven and released. Yet I felt satisfied and at peace, knowing that my heavenly Father and I knew what was going on. We shared information no one else was aware of and I knew something would eventually be done with the weights I had dropped at my Father's feet. In the same Psalm just quoted, we find this change in David's heart by the end of his cry to God,

> *"22 Cast your burden on the Lord,*
> *And He shall sustain you;*
> *He shall never permit the righteous to be moved."*

Many of the Psalms in the Bible move through this change from inward reflection and a focus on self to reflection upon God and dependence upon Him. I personally believe this happens because the writers of the Psalms were expressing their faith in God by talking with Him and sharing their deepest secrets and then the inevitable happened – God showed up!

And no wonder. Have you ever had a friend call you in the middle of the night for help? The urgent sound of their voice on the other end of the phone arrests you from your sleep and attentiveness is your natural response. We feel honored to be trusted in this way, to be awakened in the middle of the night to assist a friend through a personal dilemma. Their phone call expresses their faith in you as a friend, as a person that will not reject them, judge them, or treat them with dishonor. God feels the same way when we call on Him.

Sometimes, when I first started experiencing encounters like this with God, I would attempt to make dinner and the compulsion to overeat was not completely gone. This is because I had not yet trusted enough in God to drop all my problems, only most of them.

Besides, many of my deepest pains were still too low inside of me to reach and uncover. It was going to take a lot of time for me to find the underlying cause of my motivation for overeating each day. Yet I had seen some progress and this gave me hope for, "He who has begun a good work in you will complete it until the day of Christ Jesus."[6]

LISTEN TO HIS RESPONSE

The first part, "express our feelings about our behavior to God," cannot stand alone. If we were to carry on one-way conversations with God, we may as well be speaking to a wooden idol that is without a mouth and the ability to speak. No, our God is able to speak and desiring to speak. In fact, if we claim we cannot hear Him, we probably aren't listening. The second part to this step, **listen to His response**, is vital to the process of lasting change.

In returning to the Life Tree we talked about in Chapter Four, we see that our overeating is a fruit that has signaled to us a deeper issue in existence, lying below the surface of the soil of our Life Tree. Instead of trying to change our fruit through temporary means, such as cutting off the fruit or adopting a different set of trunk and branches (lifestyle and habits) through sheer will power and force, we must connect to the foundation of our fruit – our roots. But since our roots do not lie above ground, in our conscious, day to day thinking, we need assistance in reaching below ground to our subconscious and our past history.

Our feelings are the vehicles that bridge us to the roots of our overeating. In reviewing the soul, we remember that it is made up of our will, mind and emotions. Our roots represent our values, attitudes and beliefs. They can be found in Jesus or found in darkness, depending upon our place of deliverance in Christ. Paul actually says that we should let our roots grow down into Jesus Himself and to draw nourishment from Him. The result is growth in faith and strength.[7]

By expressing our feelings to God regarding the fruits of our lives, we now go from above ground work, to below ground work. In essence, we move from our conscious, day to day realizations, to the foundations of our thoughts, lying deeper within our subconscious. Feelings have a way of connecting us to our deeper thoughts. (See illustration next page.)

Where exactly do the roots lie within the identity of man? They lie within our hearts. Jeremiah says, "The heart is deceitful above all *things*, And desperately wicked; who can know it?" Thankfully, Jeremiah answers this question in the next verse, "I, the Lord, search the heart, I test the mind, even to give each man according to his ways, according to the **fruit** of his doings."[8] Truly God is the maker of our hearts and He is the one that understands what lies below the surface of our soil and why our fruit is yielding as it does.

So what does He usually say in times like this? In reviewing the study on our identity as triune beings in chapters 3 and 4, we are reminded that we have a choice every minute of every day to follow either our flesh or our spirit. If we come to God in a bad mood and blame outside circumstances or people, (rational as our excuses may seem) He is faithful to remind us that in Christ Jesus, we no longer can blame others for the state we are in. We can claim contentedness, joy and hope as Paul teaches us in Philippians, in all circumstances.[9] If I am having a problem keeping my joy and peace, the problem is within me.

Though this may not be an attractive answer to our problems at first, allow me to point out the hope it offers. If I am upset about how a person is treating me and I place my focus on that person, I have no control over the outcome. If, on the other hand, I place my focus upon my reaction, my resulting

Negative Behavior
CONSCIOUS
Negative Lifestyles & Habits
SADNESS
FEAR
ANGER
DISAPPOINTMENT
SUBCONSCIOUS
Negative Values
Negative Attitudes
Negative Beliefs

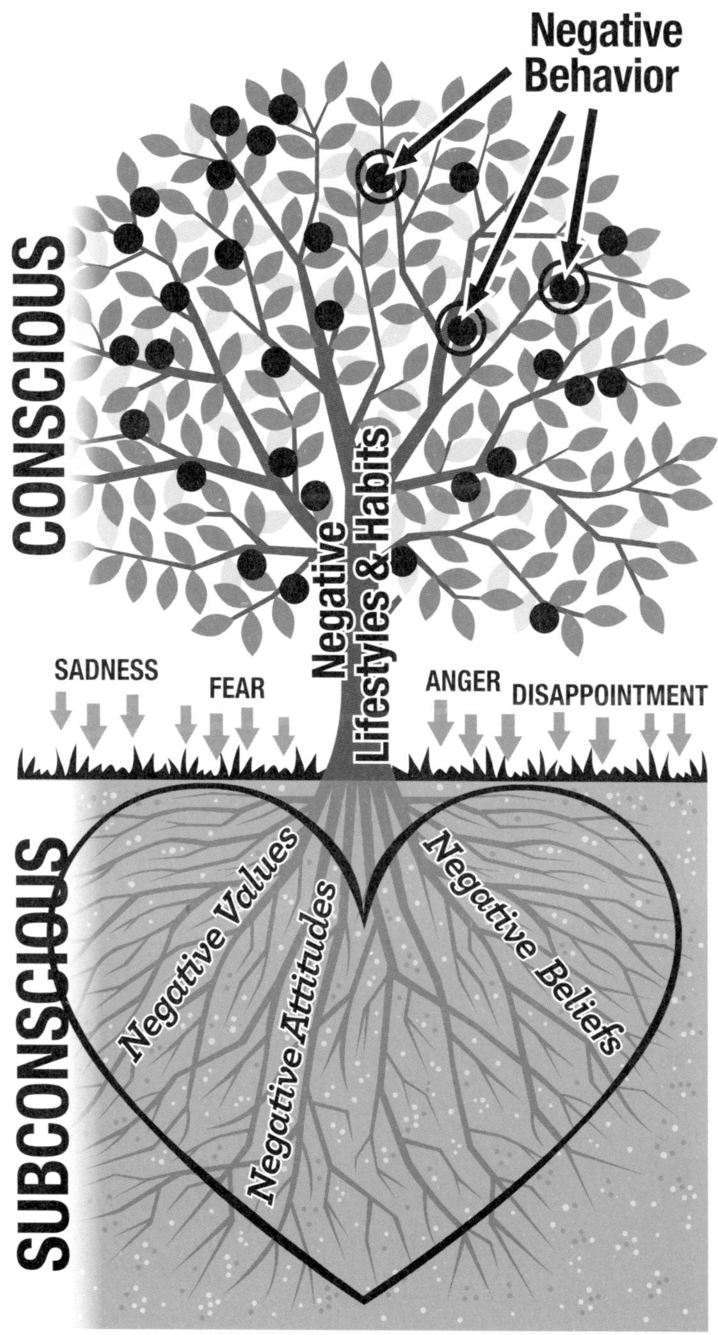

EXPRESS

thoughts and feelings, then I am in the perfect posture for change. Now I am in a posture for much hope, for God the Father can change me.

Besides, as Christians we don't have the liberty to ask God to change another person. That is manipulation and by requesting God to change a person based upon our judgments of what they need, we are, in a sense, "playing God."

No one can "make" me feel a certain way and no one can "make" me do something outside of exerted force. I choose my reactions based upon my history and my deliverance in Christ. If I react to a person with negative emotions (anger, fear, depression), I can be sure that some hidden hurt or wound is within me and I am simply reacting to a stimulant brought on by that person. There are roots to our fruit.[10]

EXPRESS

WAITING ON GOD

Five years later, as I share with God, I am still learning how to persevere in my time of sharing until every layer of fear, flesh and doubt are cut through. I can feel God, in the process, encouraging me, saying, "Do not give up, keep coming, hold on, I am almost to the center. Don't leave My presence yet."

As I resolve to stay in a state of worship, a place of waiting on Him, though I am bombarded with thoughts on what to DO, I choose to stay in a state of BEING. I don't get up from the floor, I often keep the worship music playing, I may read the Bible until I get there, but I absolutely refuse to quit until I know God and I, together, have had a breakthrough.

What a shame it would be for a person with a blockage in their heart to go through all of the physical tests, preparatory meetings, anesthesia, through the first stages of the surgery, only to be awakened with a chest wide open and told that they must get up off the surgery table to answer the phone. How is this any different from when we begin to share our hearts with God and then cut off the encounter because we think we need to call someone, or because we feel obligated to get something "important" done that day?

One sign of a breakthrough I always experience is that I have no desire to overeat. The obsession for food is completely gone. In its place there is a deep peace overriding my thoughts. Food, at this point, is supplemental. In fact, I find it hard to eat much at all after a big breakthrough with God has occurred. This place of peace can last for days. Even eating regular meals is difficult as food simply becomes something I consume in order to continue living.

Another sign of breakthrough is a shift in my focus. Like David, I usually began with specific people and circumstances that I would blame for my frustration. I could easily move into self-pity from this place of frustration but when the Holy Spirit is present, a much safer event occurs.

Instead of keeping the focus on these outside circumstances, God starts turning His finger inward at my heart and I am faced with the reality of my own selfishness, self-pity, insecurity or lack of love. Though I come to Him blaming everyone else for the state I am in, He is sure to show me my responsibility for the situation. I can tell Him all night long that my friend "made" me so angry that I had to eat ice cream. I can blame everyone else in the world for my lack of time for exercise. But in love, God redirects my focus, when I listen to His response.

This brings us to our next step in healing. Once we've expressed our feelings with God about our behavior and listened to His response, we can begin to recognize the roots of our behavior.

---

[1] Matthew Henry. *Matthew Henry's Commentary on the Bible* (Peabody, MA: Hendrickson Publishers, 1997), Matthew 26:36.

[2] "But God, who is rich in mercy, because of His great love with which He loved us, even when we were dead in trespasses, made us alive together with Christ (by grace you have been saved)," Eph. 2:4-6; "For I am persuaded that neither death nor life, nor angels nor principalities nor powers, nor things present nor things to come, nor height nor depth, nor any other created thing, shall be able to separate us from the love of God which is in Christ Jesus our Lord." Romans 8:38-39.

[3] Beth Moore. *Praying God's Word: Breaking Free from Spiritual Strongholds* (Nashville, TN: Broadman & Holman, 2000), 255.

[4] Charles Spurgeon. *Spurgeon on Prayer and Spiritual Warfare* (New Kensington, PA: Whitaker House, 1998), 135.

[5] Mark 7:14-23, Matthew 12:33-37, Luke 6:45.

[6] Philippians 1:6.

[7] Colossians 2:6-7.

[8] Jeremiah 17:9-10.

[9] Philippians 4:11-13.

[10] Matthew 12:34-35.

EXPRESS

Chapter 11

The Roots of Our Fruit

STEP 1: Release our methods of change for God's method
STEP 2: Examine a negative behavior — FRUIT
STEP 3: Express our feelings to God about our behavior and listen to His response — MOVE TO ROOTS
STEP 4: Recognize the roots of our behaviour — ROOTS

Tara came into my office with a story to tell. While running into the grocery store for a gallon of milk, she had left her younger daughter, her daughter's little friend and her teenage son in her van. As she crossed the parking lot after finishing her errand, one of her neighbors happened to walk by her. Tara kindly said, "Hello" and the woman muttered back, "I can't believe you left those babies in your car all alone."

Tara was shocked. She immediately tried to explain that her son was in the car with them and that she was only gone for a few minutes but the woman had disappeared into the store, leaving Tara alone, hurt, and without a chance to make her case.

As Tara climbed into her car, the hurt quickly turned into anger and indignation. "How could she judge me like that? Who does she think she is? I'm a good mother. How can she make that call?"

This conversation continued in her thoughts as she drove home. As soon as she was inside, she began eating all the food she could find. Her defense for being a good mother grew deeper in her mind as she stuffed herself with food until eventually she felt better ... and worse.

When I asked Tara if she understood why she had binged, she quickly said, "Yes! I know exactly why I overate! God revealed that I put too much importance in what others think of me. My reputation in the community is more important than God's perception of me. The truth is – I am a good mother! But because I reacted so badly, I guess it shows that I want everyone else to believe I'm a good mother. When they don't, I get very upset."

I couldn't have said it better myself. Instead of blaming her binge on the woman in the parking lot, she dug for the deeper reasons for her reaction. Instead of seeing every binge as someone else's fault we instead must look for the message from God.

Recognizing the root causes of our behavior is the next step toward decreasing binge eating. We must diligently seek out the deeper issues of our behavior and not get sidetracked with outward manifestations. ***If we try to decrease negative behavior by placing our focus on the behavior itself or outside sources, we will only experience temporary cures. However, if we place our focus on the root cause of our behavior, change will be lasting.***

Some of the root causes for binge behavior are sadness, rejection, fear, and confused priorities. HALT (Hungry, Angry, Lonely, Tired) is an acronym used to warn men of the preceding setting in which they find themselves most susceptible to pornography. These same conditions can set us up for overeating as well.

While working with clients, I spend a great deal of time helping them see that our meetings should not focus upon recipes, meal plans and exercise regimes. Certainly, we must become educated in these areas, but focusing only on the behavior will not bring change. The focus must always be on Jesus as the "true bread."[1] As we allow Him to become the center of our identity, He heals our hearts and we no longer need to use food for emotional comfort. Food then begins to take its God-given place as an energy source and as a part of celebration.

If you focus on results you will never change, if you focus on the God who can change you, you will get results.

I used to place the focus of my overeating on the outward symptoms. I prayed against the spirit of gluttony. I fasted and tried multiple diets and intense exercise programs, hoping they were the answer to crucifying my flesh. I blamed genetics, a slow metabolism and my hectic schedule. By focusing on the external, I failed to address the roots of my problem with overeating.

Dr. Mark Rutland talks about behavior being secondary to nature in his book, *The Finger of God*. In it, he explains that many people believe that God is holy because He does not sin. It must be understood that **because** God is holy, He does not sin. His nature of holiness **causes** his behavior to be without sin. If we counted on His ability to not sin instead of His holiness, we would be placing all the emphasis on his behavior. This would be a grave mistake.[2]

God's nature is the **source** of His behavior. We too must consider our source, our *nature,* in order to comprehend our everyday behaviors. How do we feel about ourselves? What is our identity based upon?

If Tara had blamed the woman in the parking lot for her overeating, she would not have understood why she turned to overeating. Because Tara placed her focus on the reaction she had made toward the woman in the parking lot and took ownership of how she responded, she was able to consider her own nature as the source of the problem.

Have you ever approached a weed and pulled it from its top, only to find that you left the roots in the ground? My siblings and I used to spend endless summer days weeding my mother's countless, beautiful gardens and I always wanted to get the work done quickly so I could play. My Mom demonstrated, more than once, how to pull up a weed, showing that sometimes one had to dig their fingers into the dirt to get the whole root out. Sometimes even a trowel was necessary. But I didn't like to take that extra step. I would pull on weeds from the surface of the soil, breaking the roots only partway down, if at all. I knew there were more roots in the soil. I hated knowing that I would be back at that weed in a week or so because it would quickly sprout up again.

When God pulls out the weeds of sinful behavior, He goes deep down into our hearts and tugs out every fiber, every lingering tendril of the weed in focus, until the entire plant is completely removed from the ground. Then, and only then, can that weed be declared, "dead."

Diets, exercise regimes, and appetite suppressants only cut the tops off our "weeds" of overeating. They place the emphasis on the behavior, not the nature. If you are motivated to adhere to a certain diet for a while, you may pull out only half of the roots, and then ... you know what happens. The weight comes back, the exercise ceases and your old lifestyle returns, just like the weed in the garden that grew back. We cannot force the behavior change. There is another way for it to be born. This understanding is what I call "The Fruit Principle."

THE FRUIT PRINCIPLE

If there is a tree with shallow roots, infertile soil and little exposure to the sun, a yield of fruit is not possible. This tree could command the end of its branches, "Grow, fruit! Grow, apples! Come out of my branches in Jesus' name!" But the fruit won't appear simply because of this demand. The tree could try other options. It could find a fruit-bearing tree nearby, cut a branch off and graft it into its own brittle branches. But this grafted branch would soon die. A shallow, shaded tree cannot call its own fruit into existence. Fruit is the natural byproduct of deep roots, fertile soil, and consistent sunshine and water. The results, good fruit, are promised to the tree when the tree focuses on food and nourishment.

The same is true of our lives. There is fruit of the Spirit listed in Galatians 4:20, "... love, joy, peace, patience, kindness, goodness, faithfulness, gentleness, and self-control." If I want to gain more self-control over my eating, I can't expect results by simply demanding myself to become diligent in self-control at the dinner table. I cannot "will" something to increase without feeding it properly. I do believe that there are evil spirits behind gluttony but I believe we wage 99% of the battle within our own unregenerate souls.

When I am having trouble with my eating, it is usually based on one of two reasons: 1 – there is a lack of nourishment somewhere else in my life. Or 2 – I am gaining nourishment from old roots that give me the wrong kind of supply.

If the first instance is true, I need to concentrate on letting God increase the supply. We can assist this process by practicing five Christian disciplines;

1. Reading, meditating on and memorizing God's Word,
2. Prayer,
3. Fellowship with other Christian believers,

4. Praise and worship and
5. Giving through tithes, offerings and other types of service.

These disciplines will not change your behavior in and of themselves, but they will encourage good fruit to grow.

One part of the homework my clients commit to is reading the Bible. We don't use fancy studies and special reading programs. If they have never read God's Word before I suggest they begin with the gospels in the New Testament and read one to two chapters each day. Jesus said that His "food" is to do the will of His Father. How do we come to understand our Father and the basic precepts of His will without reading His Word?

If I am gaining nourishment from old roots that give me the wrong kind of supply, I can ask God to pull out those misdirected roots and re-route them into the soil of His truth.

We need to get with God and ask, "Lord, what is behind this compulsion, this desire to eat more than I need? What is this urge in me to consume more than my body needs? Where does it come from? I need to understand the roots of this fruit."

God knows exactly what is at the root of your overeating. He knows why you opt for T.V. and internet surfing instead of exercise. He knows why you eat more bread and butter than anything else on the dinner table. He has watched you from the moment you were born and He understands all your motivations and fears.[3] Even more hopeful is that He has been waiting for you to ask Him[4] for answers because He is more interested in getting those roots pulled up than you are. AND He knows how to do it!

OVEREATERS ANONYMOUS — EMPHASIS ON A PROGRAM, NOT A PERSON

As I shared before, after graduating from college, I went into a season of great struggle. Like many that graduate with a degree but no clear plans for a career, my life seemed out of control. Public education had offered clear expectations and structure from age five to age twenty-one. I was always a "good student" and I thrived in the academic environment. Now I had to leave behind this protective cocoon and strike out on my own. I was completely at a loss as to what to do next. I had taken extra courses throughout my three and a half years in college, so I graduated a semester earlier than most of my friends. Though I thought at the time this was a wise course of action, it set me up for extra post-graduate struggle.

To make matters worse, one of my best friends died tragically in the Pan Am flight over Lockerby, Scotland. She had been in England for the semester and was flying home to New York when a bomb went off and killed every passenger aboard in mid-air.

Before this crisis hit, I had planned to move to Hilton Head Island, South Carolina to work. So after graduating in December, amidst the turmoil of my emotions, I moved away from the comfort of family and friends to face a new life of independence and freedom that I was not really ready to experience.

Making friends anywhere takes initiative and courage, but I was without either. I would come home each night to my empty, rented apartment, praying I would find a red light on my message machine, only to weep if it was black. It was during this time that I started practicing bulimic behavior full-tilt. I was vomiting, using laxatives, and exercising every day to keep my weight "under control." I also started drinking too much on the weekends and experimenting with dating as if I was taste-testing candy. In the midst of all this negative behavior, I was still reading my Bible, praying to God for help and attending church.

I can remember asking pastors and church leaders to pray for me. I believe they prayed with faith, but no one knew what to do with my eating issues. Most of these Christians were either unfamiliar with my problem or had their own problems with food.

Then I found Overeaters Anonymous (OA). I attended weekly meetings and followed an eating plan called the "Gray Sheet." I began following the "Twelve Steps" for overcoming my addiction to food. The eating plan was extremely strict. OA attendees rarely use it today but it gave me the structure I craved. I couldn't eat any sugar or white flour products and I was instructed to weigh and measure all food and drink I consumed.

I also found a sponsor to report to every day. Sponsors are people that have been successful enough in the program to help coach others along. I had to call my sponsor every morning at a specified time to report what I planned to eat that day and if I changed that plan, I was to call her and report the change.

The people in OA introduced me to the word "abstinence" and explained to me that this was to be my greatest priority in life. They taught me to count my days of abstinence and they praised me when I hit their milestone targets ... thirty days, ninety days, and one year. If I failed to strictly adhere to "the plan," I was no longer considered abstinent and I had to begin the count all over again. It was strongly suggested that I attend weekly meetings, make regular phone calls and read OA literature daily. Within the parameters of OA, I started losing weight and feeling more in control.

When I began attending OA meetings, the emphasis was on what I did instead of who I was in Christ. OA began treatment by focusing on my behavior, with the plan that the treatment would eventually move to my heart. As told by OA members, the underlying issues behind my eating disorder held the key to eliminating my overeating, but again, their schedule was abstinence first (my body's behavior) and then reconciliation of the issues (my soul). The OA program moved my focus away from God and onto my own ability to maintain control based upon dictates that were arbitrarily given to me. God wasn't the author of my abstinence and I was holding on to it with white knuckles. OA was a temporary solution, much like a diet.

Though the twelve-step program of OA is meant to lead a person to their "Higher Power," my experience fostered a dependency upon a group of equally flawed people instead of leading me to Jesus Christ as my healer. Additionally, this group of people held faith in different Higher Powers. Knowing that entirely separate theologies and lifestyles revolve around the various gods represented in one OA meeting, we were living in separate worlds. The commonality of food issues did not have the power to bring us together in unity. This only added to my struggle.

Overeaters Anonymous was a good experience on my journey to wholeness and healing but I didn't find lasting change in the program. As a Christian, I knew that God was supposed to be my primary focus, not a program and not a group of people. At that time God was teaching me the principle,

If you focus on results you will never change, if you focus on the God who can change you, you will get results.

I now realize that my loneliness while living on Hilton Head and my fear of the future were some of the root causes affecting my bulimia. It seems so obvious now. However, I could not see the core problem because I was too focused on my behavior.

As my experiences in OA attest, we must place our focus on the root causes prompting our behavior if we hope to find permanent change. There is always a stimulant and resulting reaction (Antecedent/Behavior). **Taking offense, fear, and confused priorities** are three of the most common stimulants for overeating. Another hidden culprit is **the lack of adequate rest.** Consider these stimulants as part of your personal root system. We cover them in detail in the next six chapters.

---

[1] John 6:54-58.

[2] Mark Rutland. *The Finger of God* (Anderson, IN: Bristol Books, 1988), 21-23.

[3] Psalm 139:13–16.

[4] Matthew 7:7-11.

Chapter 12

Your Journey to Healing is Unique

"For You formed my inward parts; You covered me in my mother's womb. I will praise You, for I am fearfully and wonderfully made..."[1]

Before studying the possible root causes of your behavior, keep this point in mind: there is no "one size fits all" solution in the realm of health improvement. If I were to apply a single program to the many diverse people God has created, I would be denying the unique individual histories of each person, the differing levels of readiness for change, and the distinctive physical characteristics of each person. Everyone begins at a different starting point, moves at differing speeds and struggles with a diverse set of obstacles.

As Psalm 139 above shows, God knows us very, very well. He knows exactly what we will need in our journey of releasing food as our source of comfort. Thus in my work with people who want to implement lifelong change, I place paramount emphasis on the power of the Holy Spirit to direct me in each client meeting. I also continually encourage clients to focus on God's direction and see their journey to healing as completely separate from my own journey.

Due to my past training and education, I had a tendency to try to fit all people into the same mold – the same exercise routine and diet. This is a grave mistake. As I work with an individual, we use the basic outline of my journey to healing, but we also try to remain alert to what God would have us say or do at every level. Some clients need to first learn how to rest while others need to start with exercise and proper nutrition. Nearly every client lacks some understanding in every area of health but the **order** of instruction is according to the guidance of the Holy Spirit and this is something we cannot find in a regular diet program.

Thankfully, God is not only equipped with "ears" to hear but also a "mouth" that speaks. As I meet with a client, we may have our own agendas, yet we relinquish these plans at the beginning of the hour as we pray and wait to "hear" from His wisdom the plan He has set out for our time together.

I can vividly remember one meeting where God completely re-directed my thoughts as I met with Carolyn in prayer. She and I had been discovering the connection between her loneliness and her bingeing and then tracing these feelings back to her upbringing. In the last two meetings, we were seeking healing from God for her imperfect past.

On this day I felt certain that we were to continue in this vein, but during our opening prayer, I felt moved to think upon her son, Charles. So when the timing seemed right, I asked her about her son. We then entered into a conversation about her husband and a recent conflict she had over their opposing styles of discipline. We sorted through the details and the Holy Spirit lead us to resolution in this issue. At the end, she asked me how I knew to ask about Charles, and I told her. In the silent waiting of prayer, there is much to be gained!

I believe the Lord gives us a depiction of this process in a lesson on farming in the 28th chapter of Isaiah. He explains that the cumin is scattered while the wheat is planted in rows. The farmer also processes these different grains in various but specific ways. The cumin is beaten with a stick and the wheat is ground. How to best plant and harvest these grains is direction only the Lord can give. "This also comes from the Lord of hosts, Who is wonderful in counsel and excellent in guidance."[2]

There is a basic direction to letting go of food and leaning harder upon God as our source. How we get from point A to point B will differ for each individual. Be open to His lead as you read the following chapters. Today you may hear His voice leading you out of offense. Tomorrow He may direct you to your fear of failure. Trust Him to show you the way and listen for His voice.

[1] Psalm 139: 13-16.

[2] Isaiah 28:23-29.

Chapter 13

The Root of Offense

After several years under the authority of a certain pastor, he shared that he thought I had a problem with control. He said that I showed a need to be in control of every situation, even when I was not authorized to lead. He explained that in a group situation, even if the appointed leader was not doing his or her job, I was to support and encourage them and even be willing to let things fall apart if need be, without trying to fill the void left by their lack of competence. I was not to take over. His words hit me hard. They hurt but I knew he was right. For several weeks, I lived with self-pity and remained distant from him.

Let me remind you of the battle between our flesh and spirit we considered at the beginning of this book. Accepting my pastor's accurate description of a weakness within me would cause my flesh to weaken and my spirit to gain strength. My spirit would then dictate the best response from my soul and my body's behavior would respond in like fashion.

Rejecting his assessment, I would only be feeding my flesh and starving my spirit, eventually tipping the balance of the battle for my soul in the wrong direction. At first I chose to reject his assessment. My soul at this time then dictated "death" to my body and I overate. I had taken offense and given power to my flesh, and my eating expressed this position.

After many weeks passed, I finally came to a place of submission to the truth of my pastor's words. He was right. I needed to allow others to lead me, regardless of their weaknesses. I needed to stop trying to control things that were outside of my realm of jurisdiction. Upon coming to this humbling position, my overeating due to this offense ceased.

OFFENSE

Let's now consider the following:

1. The definition of "taking offense"
2. The consequences to taking offense
3. How we can reconcile offense or avoid it altogether

THE DEFINITION OF OFFENSE

The Hebrew word, Mikshol, as used in the Old Testament is the word for "offend." It is defined as a "stumbling block, an obstacle, a cause of falling or sinning, an enticement, (especially an idol)."[1] Applying this definition, when we allow ourselves to be offended by someone else's opinions of us (whether they are accurate or not), we set up a stumbling block in our heart. In essence, their opinion becomes an idol in our mind. Contrary to God's Word, their thoughts about us replace God's truths and we thus subjugate ourselves to man's rule instead of God's.

The first time I heard that taking offense was a sin, I was listening to a sermon by Reverend Eugene Horn. He explained with scriptural references how Jesus was never offended during his life on earth. This message greatly challenged me and for the next few weeks. I found myself scanning the scriptures for a situation in which Jesus had His feelings hurt. I found none. Jesus never held man's opinion of Himself above God's. He did not hold a grudge against His accusers. He never blamed others for what happened to Him; even during His most trying times from the Garden of Gethsemane through His crucifixion on the cross.

Isaiah 53 unfolds a list of injustices suffered by Jesus, "He was led as a lamb to the slaughter, and as a sheep before its shearers is silent, so He opened not His mouth." He told us to pray for our enemies and to bless those who persecute us. He explained that forgiveness is to be practiced without limit. If we are struck on one side of our face, we are to turn to offer the other.

The sole reason why Jesus never took offense is that He walked as a complete, whole man. He never had his feelings hurt because His entire identity depended upon His Heavenly Father's thoughts toward Him. As we know, the Father was well pleased with His son. Other people's opinions about Him never swayed His own perception of Himself because He knew who He was and He knew God's plans for Him were always good. God asks us to follow Jesus' example.

Since we are not perfect as Jesus was perfect while He walked this earth, friends, family and even enemies may justifiably correct us. God uses people to speak into our lives for our own good. This was the situation with my pastor. It was possible for me to have received his correction without taking offense. I could have agreed with him humbly and asked for help with the sin of being overly dominant. I chose, instead, to reject the truth for a time and take offense, because a part of my self worth was wrapped up in my *pastor's* opinion of me, instead of God's.

Psalm 119:165, "Great peace have those who love Your law, and nothing causes them to stumble. And nothing shall offend them."

THE CONSEQUENCES OF TAKING OFFENSE

The result of taking offense is hardness of the heart. It imprisons the person offended in a place of bitterness and will eventually lead to defilement, if left unresolved.[2] By taking offense, the offended bears the burden of discomfort long after the offender has forgotten the act.

Taking offense also distances us from experiencing the love of God. In Matthew, Chapter 5, we read about offense and its consequences.

> ***"You have heard that it was said to those of old, 'You shall not murder, and whoever murders will be in danger of the judgment.' But I say to you that whoever is angry with his brother shall be in danger of the judgment. . ."[2]***

The reason I stress the importance of understanding the subject of taking offense is because I believe it is one of the most common causes behind overeating. If your spouse hurts your feelings, you may reach for an extra plate of food. Though

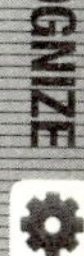

RECOGNIZE

receiving an offense may be considered an acceptable reason for eating a hot fudge sundae, as Christians, nothing can be further from the truth.

There is something incredibly deceptive about overeating when our feelings are hurt. The pain of offense seems to vanish when we eat our favorite foods. A full stomach seems to be the remedy for what ails us. Sweets or bread with butter always took the sting out of hurt for me. Yet in reality the pain had not diminished or moved, it was only suppressed. Over the years of suppression through stuffing ourselves with food, we become more and more familiar with this practice. And along with the accumulation of stuffed emotions, our body weight accumulates!

I also believe a transfer occurs when we overeat. Though we began dinner with only thoughts of our difficult day, after an uncomfortably full stomach, our thoughts shift to safer terrain such as how we are going to get this weight off. Are we going to get up early the next morning and walk or what diet can we start now? I have practiced this transfer most of my life. ***Instead of looking at what is really bothering me, I avoid it by making food and body image my main issue.***

Overeating as an answer to emotional pain can be traced back to when we were babies. When we cried, we were fed. Even if we were only crying to get love or to stop the pain of teething, our caretakers often fed us. This pattern began when we were most impressionable and for some of us, the repetition has a lasting affect.

HOW WE CAN RECONCILE OFFENSE OR AVOID IT ALTOGETHER

Is it too much to suggest that we walk as Jesus walked? Certainly not, because the Bible makes it clear that we are to live without offense.

As we covered before, our history may tell us that sugar helps inebriate emotional pain, but once we meet Jesus we are no longer bound to our history. We have a choice. We can release the pain and live life as God intended. The Word of God makes it clear that we can choose to live without taking offense.[3]

So what do we do with our hurt feelings? First, as we learned earlier – we spend time with God; express to Him our true emotions about our behavior and listen for His response. He alone can listen to every detail of our sad stories without encouraging self-pity. He will not justify retaliation, but instead will offer forgiveness, reconciliation and peace.

The second step is truly life-giving. After sharing our thoughts with God, we can ask Him to show us WHY we reacted with offense toward another person as we did. This is where things get interesting, for God knows all things. He knows the root cause of your vulnerability in this matter and merely wants you to understand your weakness as well. He knows why you were unstable in your own identity in order to take the hit. He was there when your father beat you and when your friends ridiculed or disowned you. He knows all your fragile places and He has been watching and waiting for the opportunity to heal you in each place.

He is interested in our wellbeing and will stop at nothing in order to reveal to us the root cause of our hurt within. He does this so that He can pull out the bad roots and re-direct us into the roots of His love.

Dear Heavenly Father,
In the name of Jesus Christ,
I ask You to forgive me for taking offense.
When my feelings are hurt, I recognize that I am simply reacting to old wounds and my identity is not fully founded in You. I ask You to heal me where I am wounded and forgive me for placing my identity in others. I forgive those that have wounded me and I thank You for forgiving me for my offense. Amen.

As we consider why we are hurt and how we are responsible for taking offense, we can then move to the next step in decreasing overeating (Forgive, Repent and Take Action). But before going there, we will look at three more root causes for overeating.

[1] James Stong. *The New Strong's Exhaustive Concordance* (Nashville, TN: Thomas Nelson Publishing, 1995), 78.

[2] "A brother offended is harder to win than a strong city, and contentions are like the bars of a castle." Proverbs 18:19; "Follow peace with all men, and holiness, without which no man shall see the Lord: looking diligently lest any man fail of the grace of God; lest any root of bitterness springing up trouble you, and thereby many be defiled." Hebrews 12:15.

[3] Matthew 5:21-24.

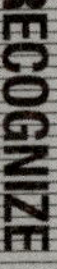

Chapter 14

The Root of Fear

Another powerful root cause for overeating is fear. As I write this chapter, I am actively facing a deep inner fear, for I have no idea what will come of these hundreds of hours of writing. I don't know the end result of this work one year from now, or how I will support myself, or where I will be working, or what direction my career in health consultation will take. While my soul (the part of me still in process of renewal) shouts that this is evidence of bad planning, my spirit (the part of me that is new, reborn) knows that it's an opportunity for living in faith.

"Now faith is the substance of things hoped for, the evidence of things not seen."[1] What does this word, *substance*, mean? The Greek word for substance in this scripture is **hupostasis**, which means "something which has been put under; therefore used for a basis or foundation, subsistence, existence; it is confidence or confident expectation."[2] So faith is something that everything else stands upon. All the writing I do and all the time and effort I put forth into this project is not solely based upon plans, budgets, people's expectations or even me. The entire structure, the process in which it moves through and the end result are all based upon faith.

It's not that I don't have plans, budgets and expectations, but even those should be established on faith. All organizational structure should be built with "spiritual flexibility," able to bend and give at any moment according to the leading of the Holy Spirit. These structures in our lives include daily schedules, monetary budgets, dietary guidelines, exercise plans, relationship boundaries, and life priorities.

Seeing a fluid organizational structure can be a little scary, especially if one has habitually learned to depend on a structure that never changes. In fact, structures that bend and flex are considered foolish in the world's view. Yet in order to live our lives in a way that reflects God's glory, we must be subject to change according to the Spirit's leading.

What does this have to do with overeating and health? Everything. Faith and health cannot be separated.

One of the reasons we subject ourselves to overindulging in food, is that we are living in fear instead of living in faith. I have noted, for the past week, that my eating has been out of control. As the week has gone by, my overeating has become worse. Now it is Saturday night. I can tell I have gained a little weight and I feel like it's only going to get worse. (If you struggle with food, you know what I am talking about – feeling like your appetite is a freight train running down an endless track.) I can't identify what is stimulating me to binge. What is the root cause to my overeating this time?

Tonight, as I was going to bed, I left my phone in my bedroom. I felt God was telling me a friend would be calling late, but He told me to answer the phone, no matter what time it was. I normally plan a 10:00 bedtime but tonight I listened to the Holy Spirit and made a small alteration. (I was about to experience the benefits of spiritual flexibility first hand.)

The call came after I had drifted into a restless sleep. While talking with my friend, he asked me how my writing had been going. He knew I had committed to writing at least two hours every day and he was holding me accountable. I started to explain all the reasons why I hadn't written for seven days and found myself becoming emotional and sad. My reasons sounded shallow and unfounded. My friend seemed to note this as well and probed me further for the roots to my procrastination.

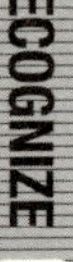

Suddenly, I saw my week's activities clearly for the first time. I had been playing a game with myself all week. I had been procrastinating and putting off what I had committed to do because I was afraid. I was afraid of writing because I didn't know the outcome of this project. The risk was too much to handle so I had busied myself with other things all week long.

As I shared this with my friend, the discomfort I had been feeling for days disappeared. It was as though I had an infection right below the surface of my skin and when my friend applied the sufficient pressure of love and truth, the infection broke. Between sobs on the phone, speaking about the fears and doubts I had been fighting, I realized that my fear of failure, my fear of the unknown and even the fear of success were causing my paralysis in writing. The subsequent dissatisfaction with myself then stimulated my desire to overeat all week. The more I procrastinated, the more I ate.

THE PARABLE OF THE SERVANTS AND TALENTS

There is a man in the Bible who also lived in fear like me. I don't know if he overate as a result of his fear, but his story will help us understand the deeper problem and solution behind fear. He is part of the parable of the servants and the talents.[3] As Jesus tells the story, a wealthy master entrusts three servants with differing amounts of talents (sums of money) as their master prepared for a long trip. The first servant received five talents, the second received two talents and the third servant received one talent. The first and second servants invested their money wisely and earned a return equal to their investments. But the third servant buried his talent in a hole for safekeeping. When the master returned, he inquired of all three servants what they had done with their talents while he was away.

The first two servants showed that they had invested their money and gained more and the master was pleased with them. This is what God calls us to do. The talents we are given include the natural abilities, character traits, and opportunities we have at our disposal. What we do with them is based upon our faith alone. It isn't what we make of our lives, it is how we live in faith with what we have been given.

When the master of the parable praises the first two servants, he describes them as "good and faithful." Good in the original Greek is the word, **agathos**, which means "profitable, useful, and benefiting others." Faithful here in the Greek is the word, **pistos**, which means "true, trustworthy, steadfast to one's promises." We are to be profitable in our time, investments, and effort in order to benefit others, including the Lord. We are to be true, trustworthy and consistent in following through with the promises we commit. The reward of these first two servants is to "enter into the joy of the Lord."

I will be the first to tell you that I lack joy in my life when I am not investing what God has given me to use for His glory. I feel listless and dissatisfied when I allow fear to rob me of my potential productivity. Eventually, overeating returns and I am left wondering what went wrong.

It's at these times that I relate to the third servant. Let's look at what happened to him. When he shared what he had done with the one talent, his master answered and said to him, "You wicked and lazy servant, you knew that I reap where I have not sown, and gather where I have not scattered seed. So you ought to have deposited my money with the bankers, and at my coming I would have received back my own with interest. Therefore take the talent from him, and give it to him who has ten talents."[4]

I used to think that this story was pretty harsh. I was sympathetic toward the third servant because I related to his fear. It concerned me that the master punished him even though he did not lose his master's money. When Jesus told parables, the kingdom of heaven and the heart of God is often revealed. What is God telling us about Himself in this story?

OUR RELATIONSHIP WITH THE MASTER

This parable's treasure lies in the role of the master. The fact that the master gave each servant a different amount, tells me that we are to focus on this initial investment and what it shows us about the master. The first two servants were given more because the master knew that they were acquainted with Him. Their relationship with their master involved love and trust. As a result, they took risk in investing but only as a response to the master's love and trust in them. Their faith was not in their own ability to invest properly, but in their master who showed he trusted them with his money! This is key to fighting fear.

In like manner, the third servant's response to the one talent investment runs parallel to his relationship with his master. Let's look closer at what he said to his master: "I knew you were a hard man, reaping where you have not sown and gathering where you have not scattered seed. And I was afraid, and went and hid your talent in the ground."[5] The servant said he knew his master as a hard man, one who didn't have his servants' best interests at heart. He didn't have a close and trusting relationship with his master and he perceived his master inaccurately. The resulting pattern of events looks like this:

NEGATIVE PERCEPTION OF MASTER =
LIVING IN FEAR OF MASTER =
AN INABILITY TO INVEST TALENTS.

Our perception of God directly affects how we live our lives. A.W. Tozer clarifies the importance of this perception of God in *The Knowledge of the Holy,*

> *"What comes into our minds when we think about God is the most important thing about us ... the most portentous fact about any man is not what he at a given time may say or do, but what he in his deep heart conceives God to be like. We tend by a secret law of the soul to move toward our mental image of God."*[6]

The third servant moved toward his mental image of God (hard and unfair) by hoarding his talent. But is God truly this way? Since the master of this parable represents God, does this mean that God changes according to how we see Him? The Bible says that God does not change. If our perception of Him is false because we lack intimacy with Him, then we may never know or experience His unchanging love for us. This is a consequence of pride. In our arrogance, we are not open to God's revelation of Himself as loving Father. Without this revelation, we, like the third servant, will be paralyzed in our potential.

Ultimately, fear's crippling effect can simply be attributed to a lack of intimacy with God. If we know Him, as the first two servants, fear will not take root in our hearts and lives. We can then gain an edge over fear and subsequently, eliminate overeating as a response to fear.

Friends and international evangelists Bill and Susan Otten, organize fear in three categories I find useful:

1. **Fear of loss** (includes lack, poverty, disease, being taken advantage of, losing family members)
2. **Fear of the unknown** (includes fear of commitment, of not being in control of our future, our children) and
3. **Fear of man** (includes rejection, failure, fear of looking stupid, fear of speaking in front of groups)

Fear can express itself through a number of negative behaviors, or even a lack of positive behaviors. Here is a list to consider:

1. **Procrastinating –** putting off activities that are difficult, foregoing actions that stretch you and your faith (fear of man and fear of the unknown)
2. **Settling for Mediocrity –** staying in a customary setting and routines to the point of boredom, lacking variety in life activities, i.e.: food eaten, type of music listened to, friendships and social events (fear of the unknown)
3. **Micromanaging –** a lack of delegation, not empowering others to take authority and responsibility but running the show yourself (fear of the unknown)
4. **Demonstrating a deficiency of ambition –** a lack in the drive to excel, to break the ceiling, to stand out in a crowd (fear of man)
5. **Hoarding –** stockpiling food in the pantry or on your dinner plate (fear of loss)

Do any of these descriptions sound familiar? If they do, fear may be limiting you in your life and it may be one of the roots to your overeating.

Eating a second portion at the dinner table may be easier than starting the business God has prompted you to begin. Waking up at night to raid the refrigerator is easier than being on your knees, weeping before God and confessing that you are afraid of your future. Eating can become a substitute behavior for what you are being asked to do by God. But God will never ask you to do more than what you and your faith are able to accomplish.

Remember,

If you focus on results you will never change, if you focus on the God who can change you, you will get results.

So if we are to decrease our fear, we need to increase our intimacy with God, allowing Him to reveal His true character to us as a loving Father. Increasing intimacy with God will occur as you go through the steps I cover in this book and we only have one more step to cover. For now, let's recognize where fear has lead to overeating and pray this prayer,

Dear Heavenly Father,
In the name of Jesus Christ, I ask You to forgive me for being afraid. I recognize that my perception of You is inaccurate and I need a change in how I see You. I want to be loosed of this fear so that I can live fully and without restraint, applying all the talents, gifts and dreams You have given me, being lead by Your Holy Spirit. I seek intimacy with You Lord. Show me the way. Thank you for forgiving me. Amen.

Now let's consider two more popular causes for overeating.

[1] Hebrews 11:1.

[2] James Strong. *The New Strong's Exhaustive Concordance* (Nashville, TN: Thomas Nelson Publishing, 1995), 94.

[3] Matthew 25:14-30.

[4] Matthew 25:26-30.

[5] Matthew 25:24-25.

[6] A. W. Tozer. *The Knowledge of the Holy* (New York, NY: Harper Collins Publishers Inc., 1961), 54.

Chapter 15

The Root of Confused Priorities

During the first appointment with my clients, I have them fill out a form called, "Priorities Exercise." It gives me a good understanding of how each person makes daily decisions in their lives. Do yourself a favor and fill it out now – it's at the end of this chapter. Be completely honest with yourself as you do the exercise and you will be in a position to learn more from the text of this chapter.

In my first meeting with Elizabeth, she claimed that she didn't have the time to exercise or prepare healthy meals. I asked her to write down all the different clubs, committees, part-time jobs, and other responsibilities that demanded time from her outside of her time with family. (Remember, this is step 2, Examine a negative behaviour.) The list was so long I was amazed that she was able to function at all each day. She was on three separate committees in her church, two civic groups in her community, and worked several part-time jobs while being a mother of two and wife of a husband that ran his own business.

For Elizabeth, this was "no big deal." She had lived most of her life this way.

For our next meeting, I asked her to write out her daily schedule for one week. I wanted to see how she juggled these responsibilities and how much time she spent on each one.

In the second meeting we had, she came to my office, flustered with embarrassment. She exclaimed, "I know exactly why I don't have time for exercise and healthy meal preparation. I do too much for everyone else!"

Once she saw on paper how busy she was, she was able to understand the reasons for her lack of health. The next step was to recognize the roots for her inability to say "no."

THE WORLD'S ORDER OF LOVE

People pleasers can be recognized as those who volunteer for the jobs no one else will do, get anxious when anyone they know is not happy, and bend over backwards to meet the demands of those around them, whether they are fair demands or not. Though it may sound like a good term by itself, no one wants to be identified as a people pleaser. The general opinion of a people pleaser is a person that does not create healthy boundaries for themselves.

As Christians, we are called to be lovers, servants of men. Yet when a person allows themselves to be stretched so thin in their capacity of serving people that their health is in jeopardy (in spirit, soul or body), there is reason to question if that person is truly living according to the perfect will of God.

Brenda admitted to me in one of our first meetings that she never reads her bible. She has been a Christian for twenty years and attends church every Sunday, raising her children in a Christian home with her Christian husband and YET, she can't remember a time where she fed off the Word of God on a regular basis for her own spiritual nourishment. She read the Bible whenever her children were responsible to study certain passages. When teaching children's church she would prepare for the classes by reading the Bible. Yet for herself, she rarely cracked open the binding.

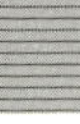

Part of the deeper root of being a people pleaser is again, that ugly word, pride. A person that wants to please others at the expense of their own health (spiritually and physically), is too dependent upon the praise and opinions of those around them. Their identity is caught up in what others think of them instead of who they are in Christ. Many mothers have a strong temptation to build their identities upon their families.

I have heard women admit, "My life is my family, that's where I find my joy." This may seem commendable at first blush but it is really out of order and even dangerous. What happens when the family disappoints them? Is their joy erased?

Oftentimes, I find that people pleasers are just lacking in experiencing the unmerited favor and love of God. Brenda believes God loves her children. She believes God will speak to them through

His Word. Even when I shared a couple examples of when God has spoken to me directly through His Word, she was perplexed and said, "I just don't know the path to where you are. I don't hear God like you do. Would He talk with me like that?"

Most of my clients fall under this descriptor. I can usually discover this aspect of their character in our first appointment by asking them to fill out the exercise you already finished at the end of this chapter.

Self Care in this exercise is not to be confused with a love for our carnal flesh, our human nature. It includes instead the stewardship of our identities in spirit, soul and body. It includes our physical, emotional, intellectual, social, financial and spiritual health. This priority includes time for healthy food preparation, time alone with God, soaking up His presence, playtime, intellectually stimulating time, exercise and sleep.

As you wrote down the order that these areas of your life take, (The Order at Present) according to importance, not according to the time you spend with each, how did that order look? I have found that most people who struggle with overeating, place "self care" in one of the bottom positions.

Renee, the client who was afraid of losing her job, struggles with finding time to exercise. She believes strongly that it is God's will that she become healthier. She is overweight and out of shape.

Renee works full-time in an office and she has a great deal of responsibility. She loves her work and has a good relationship with her boss. Yet she works overtime several days each week and she goes beyond her employer's expectations, to the demise of her health. When a fellow employee takes off for a leave of absence, Renee fills in the gap, refusing to ask for a temp employee to share the extra load. Not surprisingly, the first day we met, she filled out (The Order at Present) with herself in position five.

This may seem admirable but her goal of health conflicts with her goal of work. I liken the scenario to a soccer field in which she stands at the center with one ball. There are two goals at opposite ends of the field. At the end of a long work day, after she has done her work with excellence and her boss needs her to stay an extra two hours, she must make a choice between the two goals. One is the goal of pleasing her boss and the other is the goal of pleasing her Lord (which includes time carved out for exercise). She cannot kick to both goals. She must choose only one goal.

While describing himself and his ministry, Paul explains this choice between two masters as well, "Obviously, I'm not trying to be a people pleaser! No, I am trying to please God. If I were still trying to please people, I would not be Christ's servant."[1] (NLT) What Paul is suggesting here is that we cannot serve both God as number one and man as number one. One or the other must be the head over how I live my life. Paul reiterates this position in Colossians as well, "Whatever you do, do your work heartily, as for the Lord rather than for men, knowing that from the Lord you will receive the reward of the inheritance." [2] (NAS)

The interesting part to Brenda's scenario is that she has already won the trust and respect of her boss. She has conducted herself in the workplace with consistent excellence and loyalty. If she were to kick toward the goal of God at the end of a regular day of work, she probably wouldn't lose her employer's respect, but quite possibly gain even more.

Most people that live lives of balance get our attention. We are impressed when they leave work on the desk for the sake of family, health or church events. We are even attracted to people who leave work for parties, cultural events, hobbies and even naps. There is something quite sane and peaceful about a person that lives in such a balance. Of course, I am not talking about a lazy worker that does not earn their wages. I am talking about the smart employer that works hard, yet plays hard as well.

Consider this biblical principle,

I can only love others as I love myself and I can only love myself as God loves me.

Most Christians live life in the opposite order of this principle. They believe they can only love themselves as they love others and they can only love God as they love themselves. This is a faulty reordering of our love (others – self – God). God's order (God – self – others) is the only order that enables us to receive and then give love at a truly sacrificial, powerful level. This is why the scriptures say, "We love Him because He first loved us."[3]

God was the first to love us and He continues to be the first to reach out in love today for He is the source of all love. He embodies love. If I am not taking in love from the source of love Himself, how can I dare suggest that I am able to give love to others?[4]

I must first receive freely from God. I must first take in His love for me, His perception of me, His plan for my life. Once I take from this unlimited supply, then I can love myself and see myself as a beautiful creation, made in God's image, forgiven, washed, and acceptable. In this impartation, there comes the ability and desire to love others. It is not done out of obligation and guilt. It comes as a natural result of a life abiding in the love of my heavenly Father. We see this order of love in the following scripture,

> *"Jesus answered him, 'The first of all the commandments is: 'Hear, O Israel, the Lord our God, the Lord is one. And you shall love the Lord your God with all your heart, with all your soul, with all your mind and with all your strength. This is the first commandment. And the second, like it, is this, You shall love your neighbor as yourself. There is no other commandment greater than these.'"*[5]

This is not to say that we are to become selfish or self-centered in our love. We are told by the Bible to let nothing be done through selfish ambition or conceit, but in lowliness of mind, esteem others better than ourselves. We are not to look out only for our own interests, but also for the interests of others.[6] Yet when the order of love starts with us receiving God's love, we quickly recognize how undeserving we are of His love and in this realization, we can't help but love on others without selfish ambition or conceit. In God's order of love, selfish love is impossible! In fact, we are truly unable to carry out Jesus' instructions to love our enemies and to pray for those who persecute us unless we follow this order.[7]

What I have seen at work among people with eating problems is a lack of self care and this stems from confusion in the order of love. Without this core principle at work in a person's life, "people pleasers" don't take care of themselves and overall health continues to diminish. People are overspent and overtaxed with the burdens of those around them and are unable to continually give out without paying a price that God never asks us to pay.

I have seen ministers, teachers, mothers and caretakers of all sorts burn themselves out "working for God" because of a skewed conception of what God is like. This principle of resting in God's love first and placing their identity in Him is not known at a deep, heart level. Well-meaning fathers choose to skip family vacation in order to minister to the sick. Enlightened pastors lose track of their source of supply and become gods unto themselves and strangers in their own homes. Talented businesspeople work late and rise early only to find pneumonia and extended hospital stays barrage the end of their lives.

A seemingly good thing is not necessarily a God thing and therefore it isn't a good thing, it is sin.

Jesus did not heal all the sick. He only ministered to those the Father asked him to minister to. Jesus took trips away from His work to rest in the Father's love. He separated Himself in order to be ministered to so that He could minister to others.

Look again at this principle,

I can only love others as I love myself and I can only love myself as God loves me.

If we live with this standard guiding our lives, we will find balance and health. We will create and hold to boundaries and God will gain more glory in the end.

GOD'S ORDER OF LOVE

In revisiting the priorities exercise at the end of this chapter,

God's order begins with God in position number one. This is in line with the first and greatest commandment. In natural response to placing God first, we can see ourselves as precious in His sight and valuable in His plan so Self Care falls into position number two. In fact, love for God and Self Care practically overlap. For as we love God and obey Him fully, we are doing exactly the best we can do for ourselves. If God says we need to rest, we rest. If God says we need to work, we work. He dictates, we respond and we are provided for in all instances. Though you may think this seems hedonistic, it is quite the opposite. As I worship God throughout my existence, all that I have need of is supplied.

In reality, if God is in position number one, and we are living according to His voice, His directives, we don't really need to consider the rest of the priorities. Everything else will sit in the right place. Yet this exercise can be used as a test to see if God is truly in the number one position. Let me illustrate:

If a person places God in position number one and family in position number two and self care in position number six, my guess is that God is not truly in the first place. Sometimes this indicates that Family is in the first place.

If a person places God in position number one, work in number two and family in position three, then again, I would be lead to believe that God isn't truly in first place for God will always want our family to be a priority over our work.

Family should be in position number three. Beyond these first three, I have found that the remaining areas change in priority as life's seasons change.

I have a client that worked as an advocate for children in family court cases. Her primary role was to look out for the needs of the children and to fight for their best interest. She did this as a volunteer for many years. She loved her work and I am sure she had a positive impact on the children she represented. I cannot suggest that this work in the area, "Civic Duties" was less important than her work with her unbelieving friends or her co-workers at work or her time in church settings. Only God can direct our paths after we have made sure that He is number one in our daily priorities.

As we consider how we have ordered the priorities in our lives up to this point, how we desire to order the priorities in our lives and how God would have us live, it would be great if all three lists were the same. They rarely are. Are you pricked in your spirit? Do you want forgiveness for the mix up? Consider the following prayer:

> ***Dear Heavenly Father,***
> ***In the name of Jesus Christ, I ask You to forgive me for being a people pleaser. I ask You to forgive me for placing man above You in my life.***
>
> ***Thank You for forgiving me. I commit to the direction of the Holy Spirit now for the way in which I live. I want You to be my number one priority every day. As You live as King in my heart, I trust that I will learn to see my worth and in turn, love others as I love myself. Thank You for this miracle. Amen.***

---

[1] Galatians 1:10.

[2] Colossians 3:23-24.

[3] 1 John 4:19.

[4] 1 Thessalonians 4:9.

[5] Matthew 22:37-39.

[6] Philippians 2:3-4.

[7] Matthew 5:43-48.

Priorities Exercise

Name ______________________________ Date ____________

Civic Duties **Friends** **God**
Self Care **Family** **Work** **Church**

Write down the order that these areas of your life are in, according to importance, not according to the time you spend with each. For though God may be at a higher priority than work, I cannot make a living by reading the Bible 40 hours each week.

The Order at Present	The Order I Desire
1. ________________	1. ________________
2. ________________	2. ________________
3. ________________	3. ________________
4. ________________	4. ________________
5. ________________	5. ________________
6. ________________	6. ________________
7. ________________	7. ________________

God's Order

1. ____
2. ____
3. ____
4. ____
5. ____
6. ____
7. ____

Chapter 16

The Root of Unrest

The lack of rest in a person's life is another root supporting the bad fruit of overeating. For me personally, it's the strongest, most directly related stimulant. Looking through my years of bingeing, I see that whenever I lacked sufficient replenishment from adequate sleep, relaxation or perhaps meditation, there was the associated fruit of emotional eating. Most of my clients also lack time of restoration in their lives. In fact, I believe rest lies at the very center of health. If a person is unhealthy in spirit, soul or body, I can trace their poor health to a lack of rest, every time.

Rest allows us to fight temptation and gain victory. For it is in fatigue, anxiety, exhaustion, workaholism, and insomnia that we overeat, binge on food and quit exercise. The number one reason for a lack in exercise and a lack in the preparation and eating of whole, healthy food is "No time." And "I have too much to do, too much work!"

The worries and cares of this world war to gain control of our time and in succumbing, we lose health, we lose satisfaction, we lose life and instead, choose death.

STEPHANIE'S STORY

Stephanie was a client who had secretly suffered from bulimia for fifteen years. Her husband of over twenty years and three grown children were in the dark regarding her struggle with food. During a God-ordained lunch meeting, Stephanie asked me what I did for a living and as I shared, her eyes filled with tears. Hearing my story caused such joy in her, she was able to have hope for herself and realized that her own healing was too within reach. She knew God had brought us together at that moment in time and she was ready to reveal her "second life" so God could work through me to break her addictive cycle with food.

We worked together closely for several weeks and Stephanie was fully committed to her healing. One day she arrived to an appointment with her past week written in detail. When Stephanie and I reviewed the logging she had made regarding her behaviors, I focused on the binge/purge of Wednesday night. Then I looked at her hours of sleep leading up to that event, and I immediately saw the association between a lack of sleep and bingeing. I wondered why she wasn't getting enough sleep. As I questioned her week, the reasons rose to the top.

Two days prior to the Wednesday night binge and purge, she had less than seven hours of sleep each night. "How does that make you feel?" I asked. "Is that enough sleep?"

Her answer was immediate and resolute, "No, it's not. The biggest thing that has happened to me in the last four weeks is that I feel the effects of not enough sleep, something I had never experienced before. I now know I have to search for ways to get free time."

She continued sharing. "So at the time I kept thinking, 'How did this day go by so fast? How could I not have had enough time to do what I thought I needed to do, what I thought I wanted to do and what I thought I should do?'"

Stephanie and I slowly reconstructed the details of the day when she binged and purged, and she remembered that the battle against a binge had begun at lunch. At this point, with tears in her eyes, she shared, "Once that urge began, I had to fight all day long against it. I wondered, 'Why Lord? Why do I have to fight this battle ALL day?'"

I then asked her to tell me what happened prior to lunchtime. That morning, she went to a doctor's appointment, finished the laundry, made phone calls and emails for her growing business, and purchased the groceries for dinner and a cake. (She had promised to make a birthday cake from scratch for her sister, whose birthday party was later that evening.) When she sat down to lunch, she ate hurriedly and she ate less than she knew was nutritiously sound. She did this in an effort to compensate for the binge she knew was imminent later that evening. Amazingly enough, she had already committed to her binge in advance!

By mid-afternoon, she had made the cake and started her part-time job. Afterward she attended her daughter's dance performance *and* her sister's birthday party. By the time she arrived home, she had missed dinner and it was late. All she had eaten since lunch was a piece of that chocolate birthday cake she'd made for her sister. This set the perfect scene for a late night binge.

Does Stephanie remind you of anyone? The never-ending race against the clock. The quickly approaching deadlines. The to-do lists that are always out of reach. In other words, the angst of living without rest? The lack of rest is silent in its theft yet very threatening to our health, and it often dominates as a root cause of overeating. This is because rest is essential to our health in spirit, soul and body and without it, we suffer.

Let's consider the importance of rest and learn why it is essential to our health.

DEFINITION OF REST

There are many definitions of rest. One definition, according to Webster's, includes:

> *"...peace, ease, and refreshment as produced by sleep; repose, or a period of this..."*[1]

Rest is far more than just the sleep we get at night. But the sleep we get at night is a very good starting point.

Dr. James B. Maas, psychology professor at Cornell University, has studied and lectured on sleep since 1969. In his book, "Power Sleep,"[2] Dr. Maas gives important facts about sleep including the following:

Most people need eight to ten hours of sleep each night, but the reality is that most Americans get an average of seven hours while one third is sleeping less than six hours each night.[3]

When we choose work over sleep, we suffer the consequences. Dr. Ann McCarthy of the Institute for Traffic Safety in Albany, New York, found a nearly direct relationship between hours worked and risk of falling asleep at the wheel. Of people who worked thirty-five hours or less per week, about 20 percent reported that they had fallen asleep at the wheel; of those who worked thirty-six to forty hours,

25 percent said they had dozed off; and of the people who worked fifty or more hours per week, nearly 50 percent admitted they had fallen asleep while driving.[4]

To answer this problem of sleep deprivation, we turn to stimulants. Caffeine is the society's most acceptable drug of the 21st century. In fact, it is fashionable to invest in $5 coffees each day, buzzing around work and life on the energy this artificial stimulant offers. But caffeine is not the only stimulant we use to give us energy. We depend upon excess food to stretch our waking time as well.

Eve Van Cauter, a University of Chicago sleep researcher says that sleep deprivation causes an inability in us to curb our appetites.

Van Cauter, Director of the Research Laboratory on Sleep, Chronobiology and Neuroendocrinology at the University of Chicago School of Medicine, has spent 25 years doing research on the hormones that are affected by sleep. She says sleep deprivation activates a small part of the hypothalamus, the region of the brain that is involved in appetite regulation. She is especially intrigued by, and has done several studies on, two critical hormones involved in regulating food intake: ghrelin and leptin.[5]

These hormones influence eating in opposite ways. Ghrelin is released by the stomach and stimulates the appetite. When ghrelin levels are up, people feel hungry, Van Cauter says. On the other hand, leptin, considered a satiety or fullness hormone, is released by the fat cells and tells the brain about the current energy balance of the body.

Van Cauter examined the effect of sleep deprivation on these two hormones in her latest study, published in today's *Annals of Internal Medicine.* 12 healthy, normal-weight male volunteers, average age 22, spent time in a hospital laboratory where they ate dinner, slept, then had breakfast.

On one occasion, they were limited to four hours in bed for each of two consecutive nights. At another time, they were allowed up to 10 hours in bed for two nights. Their blood was drawn at regular intervals, and they were asked about their hunger. Findings:

- Leptin levels were 18% lower and ghrelin levels were 28% higher after they slept four hours.

- The sleep-deprived men who had the biggest hormonal changes also said they felt the most hungry and craved carbohydrate-rich foods, including cakes, candy, ice cream, pasta and bread. Those who had the smallest changes reported being the least hungry.

Several epidemiological studies show the same connection, including one from Columbia University in New York that used government data on 6,115 people to compare sleep patterns and obesity.

These researchers found that people who sleep two to four hours a night are 73% more likely to be obese than those who get seven to nine hours. Those who get five or more hours of sleep a night are 50% more likely to be obese than normal sleepers. Those who sleep six hours are 23% more likely to be obese.

And, the researchers reported, those who get 10 or more hours are 11% less likely to be obese.[6]

These results aren't surprising to me. They only support what I have found to be true in my own personal life. In fact, I believe there is a parallel between a lack of sleep and temptations to all sin (except slothfulness, of course). If we concentrated on getting enough sleep, we wouldn't have to work so hard fighting the urge to overeat. And though the idea of sleeping in may seem an easy enough answer for most of us, it's much harder than you think. It's not simply about sleeping in, or taking a power nap in the afternoon. It's about going to bed earlier, which forces us to cut back on our activities. It's also about spiritual rest, and finding that rest in God.

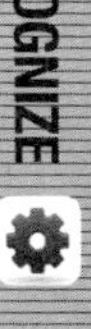

IN THE BEGINNING

God sanctified rest by resting Himself.

> *"Thus the heavens of the earth were finished and all the host of them. And on the seventh day he ended his work which he had made; and he rested on the seventh day from all his work which he had made."*[7]

Now this is important: He did not rest because He was tired. He rested as an expression of celebration, completion, satisfaction, and perhaps reflection.

The day before this day of rest, God created man. God's last day of work was man's first day of creation. Isn't that interesting? The first thing God taught man was His rest. Obviously it's pretty important.

God then instituted the command for us to rest. Rest was defined by the periods in which people did not work. The Sabbath is the seventh day, the seventh year and the fiftieth year (Jubilee). The nation of Israel was to refrain from all work during these specific days and years. This kind of rest (physical) was the only kind of rest men knew and performed because they were living according to the old Mosaic law.[8]

In some Christian groups throughout the world, rest is still performed according to a certain day of the week (Saturday or Sunday, depending on the group). Shops and businesses are closed all day, school homework is completed on the day before and even meals are made in advance so that the Sabbath only consists of worship and rest. This is an excellent practice, but there is potential danger in labeling a specific day or a specific time of the week as the chosen time for rest.

Jesus said, "The Sabbath was made for man, and not man for the Sabbath."[9] He said this to a group of Pharisees who were judging Jesus' disciples for plucking heads of grain to eat on the Sabbath. In this case, the Pharisees were placing the standard of not working on the Sabbath as more important than the needs of man. Jesus rebuked them for placing the law of rest above the law of life. We too can do this by becoming legalistic in how we practice rest. Rest is a much larger revelation than a day without work.

EXPERIENCING REST

One way I have experienced rest is simply by practicing the presence of God. It's not a time-period, but a state of being. In fact, time seems to stand still in this place of rest. I can enter into this state through worship, prayer, or simply just acknowledging God as real.

This place of rest can be experienced in activity. Though it is far more difficult to find and maintain, I can be in God's rest while I drive my car, as I wash dishes or even while I exercise. I believe it is God's will for us to constantly be in this place of rest but it is nearly impossible to practice in a time of activity without first and regularly practicing it in silent pauses.

Let's further examine how a lack of rest can encourage our bingeing.

---

[1] *Webster's New World Dictionary*, 3rd Edition (New York: Simon & Schuster, 1988), 1144.

[2] James B. Maas. *Power Sleep* (New York, New York: Harper-Collins Publishers, Inc., 1998), 45-67.

[3] National Commission of Sleep Disorders Research. *Report of the National Commission on Sleep Disorders Research*, submitted to the United States Congress and to the secretary of the U.S. Department of Health and Human Services, January 1993.

[4] Ann McCarthy, PhD. "National Forum on Sleeplessness and Crashes Staged in Washington, D.C.," the Institute for Traffic Safety in Albany, New York.

[5] Eve Van Cauter, PhD. "Leptin, Ghrelin, Hunger and Appetite during Sleep Loss," Annals of Internal Medicine 141, no 11 (7 December 2004).

[6] Nanci Hellmich. "Nightmares of too little sleep is tied to too much weight," USA Today, (November 16, 2002).

[7] Genesis 2:1.

[8] Romans 7-8.

[9] Mark 2:23-28.

Chapter 17

More on Rest

LIFE TREE

Remember the Life Tree? The fruit of the tree are the behaviors that we see evident in our lives. The trunk of the tree represents our lifestyles and habits and the roots of the tree represent mindsets, values, attitudes and beliefs. A lack of rest can be represented by the branches and trunk, for it is part of a lifestyle and it draws its nourishment from a bad set of roots.

The root thought patterns that often emanate from a lack of rest include,

"I must earn God's love."

"God will not provide for me."

"I must do it myself."

These thoughts represent mindsets fed by pride, salvation by works instead of grace, and a lack of love received from God.

As I shared in a previous chapter, I used to be a classic workaholic. I knew how to burn the candle at both ends and come up smiling. I think back to those days and they were always riddled with overeating. In my over-committed schedule, I was becoming estranged from Christ.[1] I lived by the belief that I had to earn God's love, so I was attempting to justify myself in my deeds. Yet the Bible is clear on its position of rest. Let's consider five reasons why we should rest.

REASONS WHY WE SHOULD REST

Reason #1: A Command of the Lord

The command for rest from the Lord given to the nation of Israel in the Old Testament is clear and specific,

> *"Six days you shall work, but on the seventh day you shall rest; in plowing time and in harvest you shall rest."*[2]

Behind every command of God, there is practical application. He doesn't make up rules just to see if we will obey. His rules and instructions always have substance and reason. Resting on the seventh day must have seemed impractical to the Israelites in the Old Testament. As they lived off the land, they met challenging weather patterns, failing crops, and ailing livestock. There must have been Sabbath days when rest seemed like the most absurd thing to do.

Today we too doubt the importance of rest. When circumstances tell us to press on, work harder and sleep less, we easily succumb. Yet the command for rest still speaks from the pages of the Word of God. If there was reason for rest then, we can be certain there is reason for rest now. Even if we don't understand the purpose behind the command, we need to exercise our faith in following it and we will be blessed.

Reason # 2: We are to be separate from the world.[3]

About a year ago, during a flight (from Philadelphia to Atlanta) I had a conversation with a top executive of a Fortune 500 company we will call Bill. When Bill found out what I did for a living, he shared candidly about his health problems. He admitted to a weight problem and asked me why he couldn't stop himself from late night binges and snacks.

I asked him about the time he commits to his work.

"I work extended hours all the time," he explained. "I can't think of a week in the past year that did not include overtime. But I have no choice. Now that I'm in this executive position, I have to perform at extremely high levels or I'm afraid I'll lose my job."

As I pressed him further, he admitted he felt as though he didn't deserve this job and its accompanying salary, but it was his, nonetheless. When I asked about his thoughts toward God, he said that God had, in essence, promoted him. He knew that God's favor had helped him land his position.

After we talked for these few minutes, the answer to his late night binges and obesity were obvious to me. He was suffering from a lack of rest and using food to keep his energy going. "Why don't you believe that the God who gave you this job will also help you keep this job without killing yourself at work?"

He was silent for a moment. "You're right. I don't think He will help me keep this job. I feel like I'm on my own now."

Bill's perception of God's love for him needed to expand before his waistline could diminish.

Our conversation continued as the plane landed and as we walked down the aisle and through the airport. Bill was intrigued with my assessment of his health and interested in the God I was introducing to him. He ached to know that God would provide for him even if he chose to make rest a priority in his life.

Bill is not alone. Most Americans are chained to their work yet wishing there was another way of life. Our culture encourages a rat race lifestyle. As Christians, we must live counter to our culture. We are not attracting unbelievers to our faith by living in the same work rut as the rest of the world. We must be separate from the world.

Reason #3: Faith vs. Unbelief

When we don't rest, we are expressing unbelief, self-reliance, salvation by works and any work we perform is done in vain. Basically, when we don't rest, we express a lack of faith in God and His ability or desire to provide for us. Hebrews 3 and 4 tell of the children of Israel who were not allowed to enter into God's rest. God was angry with them and said, 'They always go astray in their heart, and they have not known My ways.' So I swore in My wrath, 'They shall not enter My rest.'"[4]

And Paul follows with the instructions, "Beware, brethren, lest there be in any of you an evil heart of unbelief in departing from the living God ... And to whom did He swear that they would not enter His rest, but to those who did not obey? So we see that they could not enter in because of unbelief."[5]

Paul is referring to the unbelief that prevented the Israelites from entering into Canaan, the Promised Land. This land, in contrast to Egypt, was truly a place of rest. It was described by the Lord as "good land." This word good, in Hebrew, is the word "tov"

and it suggests favorable, joyful, convenient, fruitful. The land was also described as a "large land, flowing with milk and honey ..."[6] The bondage of hard labor suffered while under the hand of the Egyptians would be replaced by work in a fertile land where crops and livestock would multiply easily.

The Promised Land is a type and shadow of the rest we can now enter into because of Christ. It represents the spiritual and even physical inheritance we can know while living for Christ on the earth. Your Canaan can be seen in a fruitful career or business, a healthy, growing family, or even the contentedness in graduating from a University. It can stand as the small dreams and the large visions of your life. Once attaining a piece of Canaan, there is a sense of celebration and reflection, much like God's rest on the seventh day of creation.

There is, however, an inaccurate understanding of how we are to arrive in Canaan. Like the Israelites, we often live according to unbelief. We don't think God is going to provide for us so we throw ourselves into our work and cut ourselves off from society in order to meet a goal and arrive in our Canaan land. Family members, church responsibilities, and our own health are sacrificed for "promised lands" and though we do all we can to try and "make up for" these seasons of sacrifice, the time lost and the wounds of neglect run deep. God would have it differently.

If we want to live a life committed to Christ, we must sacrifice our self-reliance and become God-dependent. Recognize a lack of rest as disobedience, repent and ask God to help you find a better balance. Who better to teach you of that balance than the Son of God Himself?

Reason #4: Jesus Struck the Balance

We are to model Jesus' life and in studying Him, we see a balance between work and rest. Though He was God, he was human and He understood his limitations on earth. He was careful in how He spent His time and energy.

Author Laurie Beth Jones suggests in her book, "Jesus CEO"[7] that our Lord was a master at guarding His energy. He didn't engage in debates with those that simply wanted to argue, He didn't chase after those disinterested in His message and He encouraged His disciples to "wipe the dust from their feet"[8] when visiting towns that weren't welcoming of the gospel. If Jesus was limited as a human, we too must consider how we spend our energy. Where are our "energy leaks"? Where do we pour out effort to people contrary to God's direction? Do we even ask Him for His direction, His agenda for each day?

Not only did Jesus know how to spare His energy, but He also knew how to renew His strength. One way in which He did this was by separating Himself from the multitudes to rest and pray.

> *"And in the daytime He was teaching in the temple, but at night He went out and stayed on the mountain called Olivet. Then early in the morning all the people came to Him in the temple to hear Him."*[9]

He also invited His disciples to rest as well, "Come aside by yourselves to a deserted place and rest a while."[10]

Are we consistently reviving our source of strength with rest?

Reason #5 Love Thy Neighbor

Resting allows us to love others at a deep , authentic level. When we keep rest as a priority in our lives, we are applying the concept,

I can only love others as I love myself & I can only love myself as God loves me.

In obeying God by resting, we are allowing Him to take care of us. We are then able to give out to others by taking from the unlimited supply of our Father.

As stated in chapter 15, I must first cultivate my relationship with God. I must first take in His love for me, His perception of me,

His plan for my life. Once I take from this unlimited supply, I am full to overflowing with the ability and desire to love others. In loving God, we are refreshed enough to be refreshing to others, we are grateful enough to be gracious to others and we are rested enough to be a place of rest for others.

PRACTICAL APPLICATION

How do we know when we are working too much and resting too little? I have some tell-tale signs that can warn us of this imbalance:

1. When the priorities of God and family are not kept and our relationships with God and family members suffer because of our absence
2. When anxiety is experienced as part of our work
3. When exhaustion and then disease plague our bodies
4. When we become dependent upon caffeine, food or other drugs to keep us going
5. When we are rushed to do anything

Perhaps you are running on empty right now. Caffeine is keeping you awake, the kids are fighting for some quality time with you, sleep is something you fit in whenever you can and time alone with God happened so long ago that you don't remember it. Perhaps you are asking questions like these, 'How could I work less and still pay the bills? How can I ask for time off when the company needs me right now? When could I ever carve out time to take my wife out on a date when we barely see one another at bedtime?'

The answers to these questions depend on your faith. The God you serve is truly the God He claims to be in the Bible. He can multiply your efforts in labor today as He did for the Israelites in the Old Testament. You can separate yourself from the rat race of this world, and by God's grace, still gain favor among men and women in the workplace.

PRIORITIES AND BOUNDARIES

Are you convinced yet? Are you ready to review your hours spent each day with the guidance of the Holy Spirit?

After reflection and prayer, write out a list of time starvers. Some suggestions to what these may be follows:

1. T.V., internet surfing, reading junk mail
2. long meetings that go over the planned time
3. keeping a perfectly clean house, car, or office
4. your children's third club or activity
5. the needy person who never takes your advice and never changes
6. attending the whole party instead of half or part
7. overtime and over-demanding employers
8. controlling all facets of work instead of delegating to others

GODLY STRIVING

There is a striving in man that leads him to sin, and yet, there is a striving of God that leads to life and godliness. The Bible says we are to strive to enter into that place of rest.[11] Godly striving is inevitable because of the fight between flesh and spirit. Every day I strive for God's rest. I strive to find the time to sit, to sing, to listen to His sweet voice. I strive to separate myself, soak in a bathtub of bubbles, relax by a fire in dark woods.

He calls me throughout each day. He tells me when it's time to run away with Him. These callings may not make ordinary sense, but this is the stuff of faith.

"To this end I also labor, striving according to His working, which works in me mightily."[12]

"In returning and rest you shall be saved; in quietness and confidence shall be your strength."[13]

REVISITING STEPHANIE

Remember Stephanie? She also needs to seek out the roots to her lack of rest. We talked about the options that were available on her sister's birthday. She could have skipped both the birthday party and her daughter's performance and been home by 7:30 to eat dinner. The performance was not all that important as she has attended every one up to this point. She could have bought

her sister's cake instead of making it herself and this would have decreased her stress load.

However, she needs to understand what causes her to go the extra mile for others at the expense of her own health. I suggested to her that if all these people involved in this day, knew what she was fighting, they would be heartbroken to realize she was putting her own life at risk. Just by overextending herself she greatly increased the chance to binge and purge.

It's not selfish for her to say no. It's part of self caring. It's part of stewardship. She must place her health at a higher priority. If she assessed herself at lunchtime, when the risk level was high and she knew a red flag was going up for a binge, the conclusion regarding her day would have been simple ... it's not God's will to live this day in this way.

We have looked at many deeply rooted reasons for overeating – taking offense, fear, confusing priorities, and now rest. If you are anything like the majority of my clients, this issue of rest has been especially hard hitting. With this conviction of the Holy Spirit comes great hope! Condemnation is not in God's plan! Let's pray,

> ***Dear Heavenly Father,***
> ***in the name of Jesus Christ,***
> ***I ask You to forgive me for not resting enough. Forgive me for striving like the world, working too much and not trusting You to provide for me. I believe You will help convict me of the ways in which I disobey Your command to rest. I want to strike the balance Jesus struck in His life. Thank you for this miracle. Amen.***

With these prayers at the end of each chapter on roots for overeating, we have already begun Step #5 – Forgive, Repent and Take Action. We will dive deeper into what this means in the next chapter. With this step, these old roots can die and you can taste the freedom the Father meant for you to experience with His Son's death on the cross ...

[1] Galatians 5:1-6.

[2] Exodus 34:21.

[3] "Wherefore come out from among them, and be ye separate, saith the Lord, and touch not the unclean thing; and I will receive you, And will be a Father unto you, and ye shall be my sons and daughters, saith the Lord Almighty." (KJV) 2 Corinthians 6:17-18.

[4] Hebrews 3:10-11.

[5] Hebrews 3:12-19.

[6] Exodus 3:8.

[7] Laurie Beth Jones. *Jesus CEO Using Ancient Wisdom for Visionary Leadership* (New York, New York: Hyperion, 1995), 21-24.

[8] Matthew 10:14.

[9] Luke 21:37.

[10] Mark 6:31.

[11] Heb 4:11.

[12] Colossians 1:29.

[13] Isaiah 30:15.

Chapter 18

Lights, Camera . . . Action

STEP 1: Release our methods of change for God's method

STEP 2: Examine a negative behavior — FRUIT

STEP 3: Express our feelings to God about our behavior and listen to His response — MOVE TO ROOTS

STEP 4: Recognize the roots of our behaviour — ROOTS

STEP 5: Forgive, Repent and Take Action — TRUNK & BRANCHES

It was an interesting shift I made once I saw that unrest was the strongest cause to my overeating. I had lived my whole life believing that a hectic schedule was something to be proud of, depicting an excellent work ethic. But if the end result to this work ethic was binge eating, I had to conclude that there was something that needed to change.

Then in my quest to change I had to recognize my need to own up to this sin. I could have said that my parents brought me up this way and I can't help but work all the time. It's their fault that I strive so hard, right? I could have blamed God because it was often church work that took my time. Shifting the blame on my employers was also an option. The corporate world rewards those that "sell their souls" to the company. But in the end, I knew, I only had myself to blame.

When the Bible talks about sin, it always includes forgiveness and repentance as the mandatory response. When we uncover roots in our Life Tree that lead us to people and events in our past, as Christians, our response is simple – forgiveness. No matter who did what to us, nothing compares to Christ's forgiveness toward us and we are to follow His lead. The Christian privilege is not the liberty to do what we want, but the power to do what we ought. This power is realized in knowing Jesus and His forgiveness toward us.

The next step is in repenting for our response to how others treated us. When I first really understood repentance as God's plan to free me from binge eating, I was dumbfounded. For such a long time I had believed the lie that I was simply a victim and I was entitled to my "rightful" anger and bitter response. I ascribe this deception to the popular teachings of the 70's into which I was born. Validating emotions was an end in itself. To forgive my offenders and repent for my actions was never part of the equation. But in validated bitterness, standing without forgiveness and repentance, we find ourselves in the dead end of self pity.

Somehow we believe the lie that self pity is a comfortable place to live. And it is ... if you want to live for your flesh and not your spirit. Do you remember the study on spirit, soul, flesh and body in Chapter 4? I described the fight between flesh and spirit, saying that we can tip the scales in favor of our spirits when we feed our spirits and starve our flesh. Forgiveness and repentance will do that exactly. Humbling the soul gives life to the spirit. If you ever have the great opportunity to humble yourself, forgive and repent, it will build your spirit and increase your victory.

In *The Wounded Heart, Hope for Adult Victims of Childhood Sexual Abuse*, Dr. Dan B. Allender[1] describes this essential posture of repentance with impeccable eloquence in his chapter, *The Unlikely Route to Joy.*

> *"The primary purpose in facing victimization is not simply to know how one feels about it, but to expose more clearly the victim's subtle patterns of seeking life and comfort apart from dependence on God."*

Aha! Seeking life and comfort apart from dependence on God includes overeating, sedentary living, T.V. escapism, workaholism, sexual addiction ... the list continues. Allender calls these patterns of behavior "sinful self-protection" and he couldn't be more correct. Now we can see these behaviors as they truly are – sin, robbery, deception, death. Anything apart from faith toward God is sin. Even if our past is riddled with negative influences, we are responsible for how we live our lives today. We have a choice between death or life, worldly sorrow or godly sorrow, self-dependence or God-dependence.

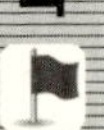

Repentance includes severe honesty, humility and at times, great grief over our own depravity. As Emily Dickinson put it,

"I like a look of Agony,
Because I know it's true —"[2]

It is only in this place of truthful self-examination that we can find hope for change. If we are committing acts of self-indulgence, seeking to protect ourselves, then we are living a lie. As God presses His finger upon behaviors that reek of self, we are more and more uncomfortable with our lie. Eventually, either we build a bigger wall around that lie or we let the impenetrable wall of self-protection come tumbling down.

Let's take the time right now to allow self-protection to die. Join with me in a prayer for forgiveness and repentance.

Dear Father, in the name of Jesus,
I come to You, recognizing my painful past,
(list those experiences that come to mind).
I choose to forgive those that have offended me.
I ask now that you forgive me for building a wall
of self-protection through the abuse of food,
sedentary living, T.V. addiction (add others that
apply). I thank You for forgiving me. I step forward
now into full repentance. I look for Your guidance
in how to move this forgiveness into action.

"If we say that we have no sin, we deceive ourselves, and the truth is not in us. If we confess our sins, He is faithful and just to forgive us our sins and to cleanse us from all unrighteousness."[3]

Repentance cannot stand on words alone. We must put our faith into action. In considering our Life Tree, we are now postured to choose the tree trunk and tree branches that produce good fruit.

Thus far we have studied our fruit, which are our behaviors. The unhealthy fruit has led us to bad roots – values, attitudes and beliefs that are rooted in our flesh. Through honest, transparent communication with God, we have come to understand these roots enough to ask God to change us, to heal us, to re-route our thinking with tendrils that are instead, covered in redemption and the life of Jesus Christ. Now we must ascend from the deep soil of our subconscious, leaving that work for God and the Holy Spirit to continue. He will direct us to further roots that need change in the future. Until then, we set out to live a life not lead by bad roots, but directed by healthy ones.

We can continue in our healing by avoiding unhealthy lifestyles and habits and choosing ones that are healthy. In behavior change terminology we say we are decreasing negative antecedents and increasing positive antecedents. Again, these are found in the trunk and branches of our Life Tree. (See illustration next page.)

DECREASING NEGATIVE ANTECEDENTS

Antecedents can be sights, smells, or sounds. They can be people or things people say. But antecedents don't have to go through one of our five senses to affect us. They can also be lies fed to us by Satan or truths spoken to us by God through the Holy Spirit.

This is the difference between external and internal antecedents. External antecedents are outside of our thoughts and are somewhat easy to control. Following are some examples.

EXTERNAL, NEGATIVE ANTECEDENTS FOR OVEREATING:

1. Glamour magazines, T.V. shows with super thin people
2. Lack of rest
3. Thirst and lack of clean, good tasting water
4. All-You-Can-Eat Buffets
5. Binge Foods in the house (that are still "forbidden")
6. Boredom and lack of productivity
7. Deprivation from food such as starvation or skipping meals
8. Deprivation from certain, enjoyable foods
9. Eating in the car or in places where you cannot enjoy your meals
10. People who steal your energy, such as those God has not called you to minister to

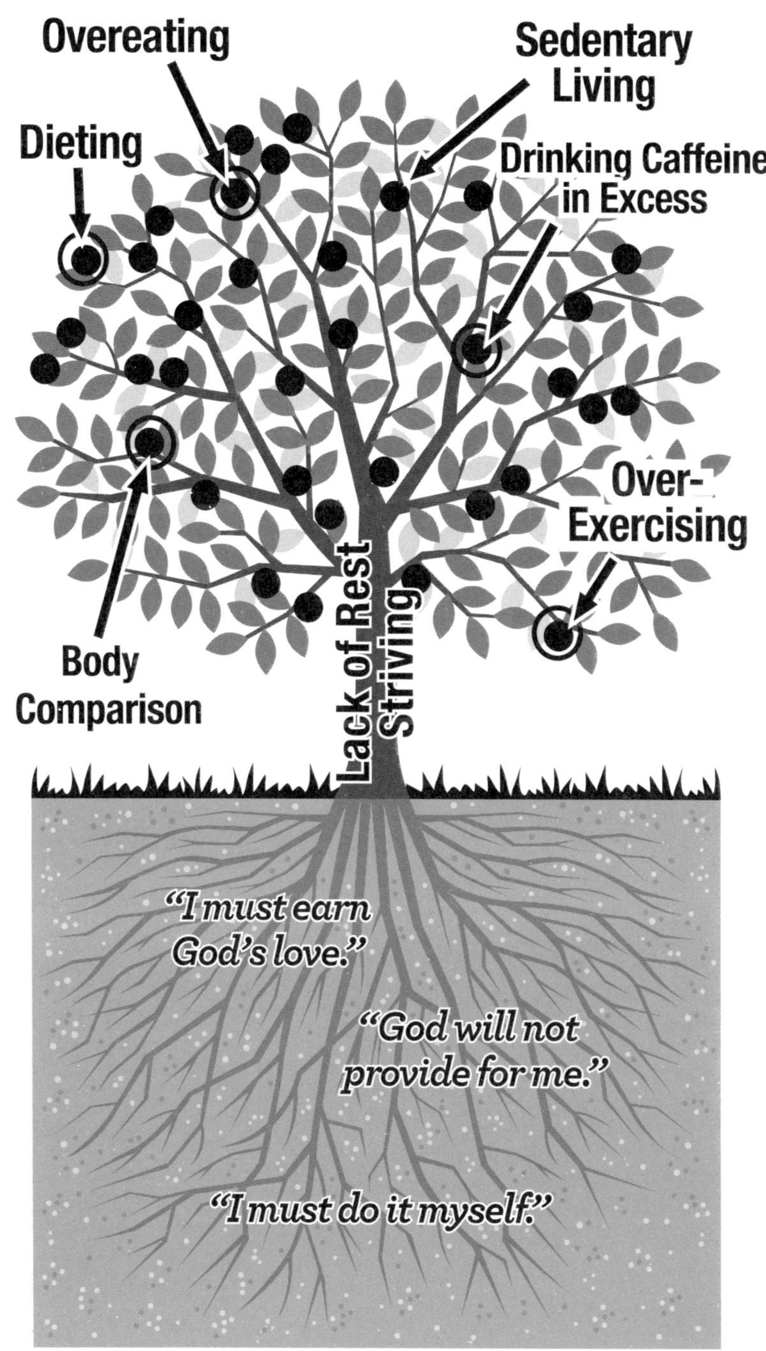

FORGIVE / REPENT

11. People who obsess about their bodies, eating and exercising or those that continually overeat and sabotage your plan for health

The following verses speak of the affect negative, external antecedents can have on our lives.

PLACES WE WANDER

In Proverbs, we read a description of a young man who placed himself in a vulnerable position for sin to enter his life. His particular temptation was adultery.

"At the window of my house I looked out through the lattice. I saw among the simple, I noticed among the young men, a youth who lacked judgment. He was going down the street near her corner, walking along in the direction of her house at twilight, as the day was fading, as the dark of night set in ..."[4]

This depiction warns us of how this man set himself up for the sin that followed. We too can set ourselves up for unhealthy behavior by placing ourselves in tempting settings. When God first began to heal me of my obsession with food, I avoided All-You-Can-Eat restaurants and I even declined invitations to parties I knew would offer large amounts of "forbidden" food. I was not strong enough yet to face the temptation of overeating. Unlike this man in Proverbs, I desired to be wise as I recognized my weaknesses before God and protected myself from unneeded struggle. This is the action that is required as the step that follows repentance.

COMPANY WE KEEP

When the nation of Israel traveled through the wilderness after leaving Egypt, the land of their captivity, they set themselves up for temptation to sin. This time it was related with whom they kept company. When they left Egypt, Exodus 12:38 says, "A mixed multitude went up with them also,"

"Now the mixed multitude (the foreign rabble) who were among them yielded to intense craving; so the children of Israel also wept again and said: 'Who will give us meat to eat? We remember the fish which we ate freely in Egypt, the cucumbers, the melons, the leeks, the onions, the garlic; but now our whole being is dried up; there is nothing at all except this manna before our eyes!"[5]

So the foreigners in the midst of Israel succumbed to complaining and the Israelites followed their lead. Who do you keep company with in life? Do they have a positive or negative impact on your eating? What if the nation of Israel had left the foreign rabble in Egypt? Who do you need to leave in your Egypt land of past gluttony?

As seen clearly in scripture, much of what our senses take in can be controlled by our environment, where we live and work and with whom we keep company. I have found that I become more obsessive about my weight and body when I spend time looking through glamour magazines. I end up comparing myself to the thin models and actors on the pages, and I then become depressed with my own body. Following this lack of acceptance of myself, I often have a tendency to skip meals or over-exercise. However, I can choose to avoid such magazines and not compare myself to the women depicted there. This is another example of decreasing external, negative antecedents.

Some external, negative antecedents are more difficult to decrease. Perhaps you have trouble with overeating when you miss regular sleep each night. If you have just given birth to a baby and your routine for sleeping and the needs of your family have greatly decreased your sleep, you may not be in the position to decrease the negative antecedent of missing sleep. But I personally believe that in such seasons of struggle, God will meet us and give us extra help. "No temptation has overtaken you except such as is common to man; but God is faithful, who will not allow you to be tempted beyond what you are able, but with the temptation will also make the way of escape, that you may be able to bear it."[6]

Decreasing negative antecedents shouldn't be confused with avoiding unpleasant but necessary situations like decreasing visits from difficult family members. If there is contention between yourself and a person God has called you to love, then there needs to be deliverance, not avoidance. Instead you need to call out for supernatural forgiveness, patience, and love.

Let's look at my previous example of overeating on Sunday nights, and see how I decreased external, negative antecedents:

1. No more heavy workloads on Mondays in order to deal with the unexpected problems that may have accumulated over the weekend
2. No more long work days – I worked 8 hours per day at maximum
3. Lunch-time breaks and 15-minute mid-afternoon breaks
4. Quitting my extra jobs teaching exercise classes in another gym and leading the Youth Group at church

Take a look at the list of external, negative antecedents I listed a few pages ago and mark the ones that affect you. Can you think of any other ones that you could commit to decreasing? Take action believing that God will help you.

INTERNAL, NEGATIVE ANTECEDENTS

We have covered external, negative antecedents extensively. Internal, negative antecedents are a different situation as they live inside of us in our values, attitudes and beliefs. They can enter our minds through suggestions made by Satan or the Holy Spirit. They are harder to recognize and control and more powerful than external antecedents. Following are some examples:

Internal, negative antecedents for overeating:

1. Negative self-talk (i.e., "God doesn't love me because I am fat.")
2. Bitterness and unforgiveness
3. Self-pity
4. Depression
5. Self-hate for one's body or appearance

I have found that these antecedents are changed not by fighting them directly, but indirectly. When light shines in our dark places, the darkness has to leave. So the way to decrease internal, negative antecedents is by increasing positive antecedents.

PRAYING FOR AND PLANNING FOR POSITIVE ANTECEDENTS

Positive antecedents are the stimulants that boost our success in decreasing unhealthy habits or increasing healthy habits. They help motivate us to do what is right. Again, external antecedents are the ones that we can easily control because they are on the "outside."

Following are some external, positive antecedents in the case of overeating:

1. Keeping fresh fruit and vegetables readily available
2. Buying cookbooks that stress healthy and flavorful cooking.
3. Keeping water in abundance wherever you go
4. Finding restaurants that offer healthy meals
5. Ordering your life around specific meal times every day, especially weekends
6. Keeping meal replacements handy in case there is no time for a meal
7. Taking 15-minute breaks while at work to refresh oneself
8. Dinner time is often the most difficult time for overeaters. I believe that the stress of the day and the fatigue caused by activity and challenges can increase the chances for overeating. I have found that just having some kind of plan for the time after dinner will help stop the craving for the second portion.

Here are some examples of external, positive antecedents in the case of exercise:

1. Listening to great music while walking
2. Establishing a routine time for working out
3. Staying accountable to exercise by having a workout partner
4. Using variety so that boredom of the activity does not set in
5. Finding enjoyable surroundings to exercise in
6. Finding convenient places to exercise
7. Choosing comfortable movement (as comfortable as we can get it)
8. Wearing comfortable, sturdy shoes and flattering clothes while exercising

The five basic key habits for Christian living covered in Chapter 11 will allow the Holy Spirit to transform us and they concentrate on **internal** change. These positive, internal antecedents are 1) reading, meditating on and memorizing God's Word,

2) prayer, 3) fellowship with other Christian believers, 4) praise and worship and 5) giving through tithes, offerings and other types of service. These habits allow our tree to live and grow good fruit.

The Bible explains that we are transformed when our minds are renewed and we are renewed by the word of God.[7] It also says that we are renewed as we gain knowledge of our Creator.[8] This knowledge comes from receiving God's revelatory word (rhema), which is increased as we spend time with God and by reading His written word (graphe) and gaining in the meaning of the word (logos). Reading the Bible and prayer go hand in hand and are essential to victory against sin.

Fellowshipping with other believers is also key to the renewing of our minds. Spending time in praise and worship is another supernatural method that recharges our spiritual batteries. Giving then causes us to live extended to others. It pulls us from isolation to responsibility.

I have a client who has been working diligently through the steps of change outlined in this book. She believes in Jesus, attends church, and is beginning to dig into a deeper place of intimacy with God. The bad roots to her eating binges are being exposed and she is processing everything with great courage and transparency. Her eating binges have decreased measurably. However, a choice arises as the buffer of food continues to decrease.

There is a danger to getting to this place of root exposure without basic Christian disciplines in constant, daily practice. Every day, the world and its philosophies are offered as solutions to her pain. She could begin to lean upon other people that do not lead her to God, she could find herself attracted to unhealthy relationships, or even substitute addictions. The Christian disciplines of reading the Bible, prayer, worship, fellowship and service to others will give her the boundaries, structure and outline for living that will keep her from such danger. They will also keep the channels of communication open between herself and God so that she can hear clearly as He speaks to the specific areas of woundedness that He desires to heal.

REVISIT RENEE

We have now arrived at the end of the five steps that lead us to a healing of food dependence. As a review, let's apply these five steps of change to Renee, the client that had trouble leaving work on time.

Step #1 — She must first release her will for God's will, no matter what it may be, avoiding fad diets and expensive gym memberships she won't use.

Step #2 — She next examines her behavior and finds that she doesn't have time for exercise or healthy meal planning because she works overtime at the office most days.

Step #3 — She spends time with God, talking about her overworking and listening to His response.

Step #4 — God responds by telling her that he loves her and that overworking is not in His plan for her life. This step causes her to dig down to the root problem and recognize why she has a mindset that causes her to want to earn the admiration of her boss through extra effort. Why does she choose him over her own health? Has she always placed others over herself? Why isn't she striving to find God's rest? What is it about making healthy boundaries for herself that is so unattractive to her? As the roots are revealed, she forgives all the people that are involved and she moves to repentance.

Step #5 — Once God reveals the roots of her behavior and repentance has taken place, there needs to be action that follows the faith. She meets with her boss and explains that she will not be taking up the slack of other employees and that she will be endeavoring to leave on time every day.

By the way, sometimes more of the bad roots appear once Step #5 takes place. If Renee goes against her feelings and fears and actually leaves work at quitting time, trusting God to fill in the gaps she has left, she may get in touch with more deep feelings. Roots such as shame and guilt may increase. She is then to go back to Step #4 and work with God on the root reasons for her negative feelings.

Perhaps she connects these feelings to how her father used to treat her when her effort was less than 110%. Then she needs to repent for living for her father's affirmation instead of God's and continue to act out her faith in God, trusting Him to give her favor with Himself and with man, in due time.

As Renee continues to practice these 5 steps, she begins to experience a miracle. She has more excitement about her life. She believes that God is her provider and she finds that instead of losing the favor of her boss, he is now hiring an additional employee to help out with the office workload. God then blesses the boss with more work because He favors Renee's choices of obeying Him. Renee is now making time for exercise and planning healthy meals. She is losing weight but the real miracle is that she is no longer a door mat and the Director of her life is the Creator of the Universe, not her boss (or her father incarnate). God is loving on Renee and, as a result, her understanding of her worth is increasing and the cycle continues.

We are now nearing the end of the healing process. Behavior has been covered in great depth. Now we conclude by considering two more parts of behavior change theory – rewards and consequences. Though these two parts of change have been given great credit in the history of human behavior change, I have put them up against the Bible and found startling results. Let's look at the "Ultimate Behaviorist's" viewpoint of rewards and consequences in the next two chapters.

---

[1] Dan B. Allender, PhD. *The Wounded Heart, Hope for Adult Victims of Childhood Sexual Abuse*, (Colorado Springs, CO: NavPress, 1990), 177.

[2] E. Dickinson. *The Poems of Emily Dickinson*, 339 (Boston, MA: Little, Brown and Company, 1890), 152.

[3] 1 John 1:8-9.

[4] Proverbs 7:6-27.

[5] Numbers 11:4.

[6] 1 Corinthians 10:13.

[7] Romans 12:1-2.

[8] Colossians 3:10.

Chapter 19

Our Great Reward

I grew up on a farm in upstate New York and my parents didn't give me rewards for doing daily chores, which was a wise decision on their part. I milked goats morning and night throughout my middle school and high school years. When the snow was up to my knees and the hairs in my nostrils would freeze upon stepping outside of the house, going to the barn to milk was the last chore I wanted to do. I can remember running full tilt from the porch to the barn counting the strides I made, the silver milk bucket hooked in my arm, clanging against me. Entering the barn, the smell of old hay and the mooing of cows waiting for their meal would fill my senses. As I pressed my head to the warm belly of Sally, our goat, and watched the steam float up from the pail of fresh milk, I would enter into a restful state.

I may not have understood it fully at the time, but there was reward within the farm chores I completed every day. I was gaining confidence in myself as I was entrusted with these farm animals' well being. I found joy and contentedness in the quiet of the barn. And I experienced a sense of success in bringing that full pail of milk into the house for our family to consume.

I'm certain there is even greater reward today as I glean from those years of farm work in my ability to perform a task to completion, on time, consistent, every day.

In most behavior change models, rewards are considered an essential part. They can be intrinsic or extrinsic. **Extrinsic rewards** are incentives planned out by a person to increase the motivation for change. Buying new clothes when we reach a certain weight goal and booking massages or vacations are examples of extrinsic rewards suggested by many diet programs. Behavior change theory places great emphasis on the planning of extrinsic rewards when we are trying to adopt positive behavior.

Concerning weight loss, I know that extrinsic rewards do not work. When I first started coaching people in pursuing lifetime change, extrinsic rewards never showed great results. I would encourage clients to set up massage appointments, special events or just shopping sprees in advance of meeting certain goals. Rarely did a client seem comfortable in even planning special treats, let alone in following through with applying them when they met their personal objectives.

Part of the problem lies in the fact that most people struggling with emotional eating do not feel they deserve special treats. The Priorities Exercise we do together in our first meeting fleshes out a low sense of self worth as they place "Self Care" in one of the last positions, under family, friends, church and work. However, low self worth is only part of the problem. There is a deeper reason for the ineffectiveness of planned extrinsic rewards. The power of incentives is not fully realized until a person discovers intrinsic rewards.

Intrinsic rewards, as the term suggests, come from within. Examples include increased self-esteem, joy, peace and love for myself and others. Intrinsic rewards are the more powerful of the two types of rewards though they cannot be directly controlled or planned out. They come as byproducts of positive behavior, much like the good feelings I'd experienced when doing farm chores. Following the plan of health outlined in these chapters, we take the emphasis off extrinsic rewards and harness the power of intrinsic rewards instead. We do this in an unexpected way, **by ignoring both.**

FOR THE BIBLE TELLS ME SO

God is the giver of both intrinsic and extrinsic rewards. James tells us that every good gift is from God.[1] Jesus says that family, houses, fields and eternal life are promised to those that sacrifice earthly gain for His kingdom.[2] In the book of Hebrews, the writer says that God rewards those who sincerely seek Him.[3] Revelations quotes Jesus as saying that His reward is coming and is found in Him.[4] When Paul speaks of running the race of life in faith, he speaks of a "crown that will last forever" and a prize that is worth every bit of strain and effort.[5]

Since God is the giver of all good rewards, why should we seek them out ourselves? We need only seek after Him and we get all the rewards we could desire.

If you focus on results (rewards) you will never change, if you focus on the God who can change you, you will get results (rewards).

I used to focus on the rewards I could gain – a thinner body, peace with food, answers to my bingeing. When God shifted my focus to Him, intimacy with Him increased. In direct response to this increased intimacy, I started experiencing both the extrinsic and intrinsic rewards I used to seek – weight loss, an increase in energy, an increase in self-esteem. Yet the reward of God Himself had to come first.

Mike Bickel, founder of the International House of Prayer in Kansas City, agrees,

"God revealed Himself as the primary reward of the human heart in Genesis 15:1 when He stood before Abraham and said, 'Do not be afraid, Abram. I am your shield, your exceedingly great reward.' Those words amaze me. God reveals Himself as our prize. He is the ultimate satisfaction of our hearts. He gives us secondary rewards, too, and I love them as well. There's the anointing to touch the ends of the earth. There's health, wealth and influence, anointed ministry and favor in significant relationships. God gave all of these to Abraham and promised them to us. But they are all secondary. God Himself was the great reward surpassing all others. He is the prize of the ages."[6]

I can now agree with the writer of Lamentations in saying, "'The LORD is my portion', says my soul, 'Therefore I hope in Him!'"[7]

It's tempting to seek rewards other than Jesus. All too often, we were brought up looking for these kinds of rewards. Many people raise their children this way today. Instead of allowing God to bring about the intrinsic and extrinsic rewards of positive behavior, we contrive rewards by offering money (or worse, candy or ice cream) when a child follows through with a responsibility. This creates a false sense of security in rewards. I believe that children need to learn at an early age that rewards don't always come as we expect them and they are oftentimes delayed.

DELAYED GRATIFICATION

Scott M. Peck introduced me to delayed gratification in his book, *The Road Less Traveled.*[8] He explains that the time we spend waiting before we realize a reward matures us and causes us to place more emphasis on the process of change instead of the result.

What happens when rewards are delayed? How do we continue to exercise and eat healthfully when we do not see weight loss? First of all, this question reveals that the reward we seek is the wrong one. In Philip Yancey's book, *Where is God When It Hurts?*[9] he explains how Job's faith was not based upon worldly rewards.

Yancey says, "In the first two chapters of Job, Satan reveals himself as the first great behaviorist. He claimed that faith is merely a product of environment and circumstances. Job was conditioned to love God. Take away the positive rewards, Satan challenged, and watch Job's faith crumble."

As we know, Job's faith in God stood strong even without worldly reward. His faith in God was not dependent upon outside circumstance. We too must be sure that our faith in God is not dependent upon weight loss, a smaller dress size or disease-free living. If our faith increased toward God because of weight loss, then what happens if we gain the weight back? It's dangerous to place emphasis on these kinds of rewards. Worldly rewards change and we really don't have much control over them.

Delayed rewards are also teachers in our process of maturity. The cycle of life is punctuated with seasons of sowing and reaping. In the seasons of sowing, there is little tangible reward.

"Do not be deceived: God cannot be mocked. A man reaps what he sows. The one who sows to please his sinful nature, from that nature will reap destruction; the one who sows to please the

Spirit, from the Spirit will reap eternal life. Let us not become weary in doing good, for at the proper time we will reap a harvest if we do not give up."[10]

At the proper time, we will gain reward. Yet, in the meantime the only reward we may find from hard work is the sense of accomplishment alone. The season of reaping has not yet come. Though the tangible reward is not seen (increased energy, peace with food, weight loss, lower blood pressure, muscle strength), the behavior is still positive. We may be conditioned to expect immediate rewards and lose patience and fail to persevere when in the season of sowing. However, this response expresses confusion in the one great reward – God Himself.

APPLICATION

There was a time when I struggled with my boss at work. For whatever reason, she didn't delegate new responsibilities to me, even though I felt I was capable of handling more work. I became bored with my job. I went to work dreading the lack of challenges that awaited me. For a time I created projects on my own, trying to stay busy. Yet this didn't satisfy. I was angry with my boss, I felt inferior and unimportant. In my frustration, I would overeat to deal with my feelings. When I prayed about it, I knew God didn't want me to leave this job. So I started tackling this issue with God at home, telling Him my feelings, crying out to Him about my pain and frustration.

In those times, it became quickly evident that I had within me a deeper need to feel validated and important. I wanted to be esteemed by people through an increase in my responsibilities and a title of prestige. God then showed me that I was to be content serving my boss and content to do everything she gave me and to do it with excellence. The Lord was to be my focus and my only judge and employer. He was also to be my reward. I was to be content in serving Him by serving my boss.

He talked with me about waiting on Him for all things and trusting His timing. He showed me verses of scripture such as "Let not mercy and truth forsake you; bind them around your neck, write them on the tablet of your heart, **and so find favor and high esteem in the sight of God and man.**"[11] I also related well with David as he served Saul, knowing that God had anointed David to be king. But David stayed in the cave of Adullam and allowed God to train him in serving and waiting. [12]

I started repenting for my wrong attitude of superiority and I prayed for my boss. I learned to bite my tongue and support her in all her efforts and allow all accolades to go to her. I worked hard with all she gave me and concentrated on producing excellent products, on time, every time. It was never easy. I had to fight bitterness all the way. I had to be on guard against Satan who wanted to rob me of joy in the workplace. I kept God's Word close to my heart and depended upon Him to come through for me. He definitely came through. My overeating decreased as a result.

I stayed in that job for three years. If anyone had told me at the start that it would be that long, I would have left. Yet in that period, God proved sovereign. I earned my master's degree with the extra time I had and I learned a lot about serving people and waiting on God. I was later promoted to the position my former boss held and served in that capacity for two years. I also had learned an invaluable lesson about the importance of delegation. From the day I started to the day I left that position, I delegated responsibilities to my employees to help them develop in all the areas in which they showed interest. I found out that I was still in a capacity of serving people but it was wonderful to see the fruit of higher self-esteem and lessons learned as they worked with the challenges I gave them.

None of this growth and experience would have occurred if food had not served as a signal of something wrong in my heart. If I hadn't expressed my feelings with God and heard His voice concerning the greater issues lying in my heart, I would have never passed this test. As I followed His will with repentance and faith, He took those three years and blessed me abundantly. Yet the blessings, the rewards were not simply found in weight loss, my promotion, in my furthered education or even in the lesson I learned about delegation. The reward I found was God Himself. Other rewards came as bonuses.

[1] James 1:17.

[2] Matthew 19:29.

[3] Hebrews 11:6.

[4] Revelations 22:12.

[5] 1 Corinthians 9:24-27.

[6] Mike Bickle. *Song of Songs: The Ravished Heart of God with Mike Bickle, CD Session 7* (Kansas City, MO: Friends of the Bridegroom, 1999).

[7] Lamentations 3:24.

[8] Scott M. Peck. *The Road Less Traveled* (New York, NY : Touchstone, 1978), 18-20

[9] Philip Yancey. *Where is God When It Hurts?* (Grand Rapids, MI: Zondervan, 1990), 105.

[10] Galatians 6:7-9.

[11] Proverbs 3:1-4.

[12] 1 Samuel 24.

Chapter 20

The Gift of Consequences

We have now arrived at the end of Behavior Change Theory with "Consequences" or the results of our behavior. Consequences can be positive or negative.

In our culture, the word "consequence" only carries a negative connotation. Yet consequences of negative behavior are often the catalysts for positive, lasting change.

Pain is a powerful consequence and Philip Yancey explains its importance in his book, "Where is God When It Hurts."[1] He emphasizes the value of pain in his study of lepers. Widely misunderstood, leprosy is a disease of the nervous system and lepers inflict wounds upon themselves without knowing it because the sensation of pain is not present in their extremities. Lepers are fitted with special shoes and gloves to help them realize more quickly that they may be stubbing their toes or damaging their fingers in everyday activities. Perhaps you don't struggle with this disease but we become "spiritual lepers" when we dodge pain by using drugs, overly busy schedules, overeating and other tools of avoidance. This is a more serious disease than leprosy as it is a disease that affects your spiritual victory.

If, for example, a person overeats for a number of months and then finds that the waistline of their clothes is too snug, the consequence of having to go shopping and buy new pants may be a motivational factor in getting the person to cut back on calories consumed. The feelings of disappointment, sadness, and dissatisfaction in the way clothes fit could actually help cause a positive reaction.

In not wanting to face up to the reality of our behaviors and the painful results of bad habits, we often find ways to "hide" the behaviors' results. A person who overeats during the weekend could choose to avoid the consequence of a tight waistline by skipping breakfast and lunch during the following week. This may seem like a wise choice to the person at the time, but in reality, this way of avoiding consequences can be more like personal sabotage.

Skipping breakfast and lunch is an unhealthy habit and though short-term weight loss may be achieved, metabolism is slowed down and energy becomes inconsistent throughout the day because of the limited energy source from only eating dinner. Besides, this habit of skipping meals during the week may set a person up for bingeing and therefore only fuel the original behavior of overeating during the weekend. If instead, the person were to accept the consequence of a tight waistline and experience the fear of needing new clothes, motivation may increase for changing the habit of overeating during the weekend.

So consequences can be something quite valuable. They teach us about the positive or negative fruit of chosen behavior. The more directly related a consequence is to the behavior, the stronger the lesson will be and therefore, the stronger the motivation to change. Other examples of consequence avoidance for weight gain are:

1. over exercising that compensates for overeating
2. choosing pants and skirts with elastic waistlines over ones with buttoned or zippered waistlines
3. avoiding all bread, potatoes, pasta and cereal to lose water weight
4. avoiding intimacy with a spouse or keeping "hidden" from a spouse during intimate moments
5. staying away from public events or events where regular attire is bathing suits
6. shying away from the camera for pictures or standing in the back, behind others
7. not trying on bathing suits in the store
8. avoiding full-length mirrors

These are methods used to avoid the consequences of overeating. Similarly, there are avoidance techniques for **all** unhealthy behaviors.

Medications are another way we avoid consequences. If I don't drink water all day and become dehydrated and then experience a headache, I can reach for pain reliever. This pain reliever, in essence, stops me from experiencing a consequence that could teach me a lesson and help me change my behavior of dehydrating myself.

Food and overeating are often used to push down and anesthetize pain. Instead of experiencing the suffering of daily life and crying in the arms of our Lord, we stuff our emotions down with food. I am convinced that this is the number one reason why people overeat in the evening. Night-time is a time in which all the struggles and issues of the day come before us for review. Our bodies are often exhausted, our emotions are frazzled and we are brought to a place of rest, at least a type of rest that is different from the constant, active "buzz" of the work day. So we avoid reviewing the day's triumphs and defeats by engaging in behavior that prompts escape like watching T.V., drinking alcohol, or eating excessive food.

Try as we may to stop the consequences of our negative behavior from becoming evident, this battle is futile for consequences are imminent. In fact, I believe they are built up through time. This is why we get heavier and heavier with age. This is why the aspirin we take for a headache caused by dehydration soon becomes prescription medication for migraines which then wreak havoc on our bodies with their side effects, all the while the body is crying simply for more water.

We often do the same in rearing our children. Instead of allowing consequences to teach them that their behaviors are negative, we console and even at times, buffer the consequences so that pain will not be experienced by our children. Yet it is in the consequences that we can gain insight that spurs change. Paul writes of this phenomenon as he addresses the Corinthians, "... if I made you sorry with my letter, I do not regret it; though I did regret it. For I perceive that the same epistle made you sorry, but that your sorrow led to repentance."[2]

God works in the positive consequences of life. But more often than we realize, He's at work during the negative ones too. "And not only that, but we also glory in tribulations, knowing that tribulation produces perseverance; and perseverance, character; and character, hope." Romans 5:3

Consequences that may encourage a person to positive change:

1. Weigh yourself once each week or perhaps even once each day
2. Take girth measurements in hips, abdomen and thighs once each week
3. Take a full-length picture of yourself in a bathing suit (or without)
4. Get screenings for blood pressure, cholesterol, and cardiovascular strength (stress test)
5. Log the food and beverages consumed with accuracy

As we trust negative consequences to do a work in us that continues us toward health and decreased overeating, let's now consider one last part to behavior change that is deceptively empty – Maintenance.

---

[1] Philip Yancey. *Where is God When It Hurts?* (Grand Rapids, MI: Zondervan, 1990), 32-33.

[2] 2 Corinthians 7:8.

Chapter 21

The Faulty Concept of Maintenance

Maintenance is not a biblical word, really. God never asks us to maintain our spiritual faith and stay satisfied with our present state. He is always pressing us further into Him. He is always maturing us and leading us to higher levels of faith, love and good deeds. When one area of our lives seems stronger and more Christ-like, God is there to kindly present the next place in our hearts that needs to be changed.[1]

Eustress is a positive form of stress that researchers have deemed essential to satisfaction in life. It is the stress that gets your blood pumping without nearing the boiling point.

Without this kind of stress, we lose the zest that life offers. We start to draw inward and can become depressed. You have probably experienced this phenomenon after finishing a big project or being in a large production of some sort. Even the letdown after the holidays can take us to this lonely place.

I have a good friend that competes in triathlons and Ironman events. I recently talked with him after a long and successful race and he candidly admitted to feelings of depression after he crossed the finish line. He had trained and worked hard for months for that one-day event and now that it was over, what was next? Perhaps he was putting too much faith in that one event and the perceived satisfaction that would follow in reaching that single level of racing success. But the truth is,

There is no such thing as maintenance in the kingdom of God.

Belief in the concept of maintenance is the main reason why diets fail. We can take the weight off, but keeping it off is another story. This is because maintenance is a faulty concept. After a person reaches a certain goal weight, they rarely have the next goal in sight. They try to move into the stage of maintenance. Yet I don't think maintenance is actually possible for humans for we were created to strive for the next goal. By God's divine plan, we are called to the next challenge. Step by step, level by level, we are beckoned to move further along the continuum, in the process of maturity, in the attainment of greater health in all areas of our lives.

GOAL SETTING

I once heard an athletic coach explain the importance of goals. He said that once you have attained a goal, you must be quick to set the next goal or you will become complacent, and will eventually start to move backwards. God has made us as human beings who love a challenge. We were created to pursue places of higher excellence in all areas of our lives. There is within us a joy, a satisfaction in facing a struggle and winning the battles of life which bring excitement and purpose to our lives (eustress). They help us focus our energies and they trigger us to pull from our deepest potentials. Consider Paul's excitement as he speaks of the pressing he does toward the goal of his life,

"I keep working toward that day when I will finally be all that Christ Jesus saved me for and wants me to be. No, dear brothers and sisters, I am still not all I should be, but I am focusing all my energies on this one thing: Forgetting the past and looking forward to what lies ahead, I strain to reach the end of the race and receive the prize for which God, through Christ Jesus, is calling us up to heaven."[2]

In presenting a case against maintenance, I'm not saying that we have to continue losing weight, as this would be impossible. Instead, God may have other goals in mind for me. Once I reach my goal weight I may then receive conviction from God regarding my intake of caffeine (not until this book is done!). Or perhaps my next health goal is to decrease processed foods to one meal each day.

When I first realized that the concept of maintenance is not in the kingdom of God, I feared I would gain back the weight I lost. But God's method for increased health has a built-in guarantee that keeps me growing in my new found healing. It's what some may call "discipling," and I believe it is God's answer to the world's concept of maintenance.

MAKING DISCIPLES

Since my healing from the bondage of food first began, I have had continual opportunity to share the hope He has given me with others that struggle with food. As I mentioned before, as soon as I began this journey toward releasing food and depending upon God, I had my first "converts" knocking at my door. I didn't have a whole lot to give them, but what I did have, I gave freely. In doing this, I was encouraged in my own growth and by leading others, I was motivated to find new ways of sharing the miracle of healing that had been given to me. My writing increased, I spoke at Christian meetings and I did a series of presentations on the definition of "rest."

Most of my clients have found similar opportunities to share with others. And it isn't something we have planned. God brings these people into our sphere of influence. As soon as we have something good to give, God chooses to grow our faith by causing us to pass it on.

This is the great commission, "Therefore, go and make disciples of all the nations, ..."[3] At first this looks like a command to sell our worldly possessions and live in grass huts as missionaries in Africa. I have realized instead that my unreached nation dwells within the two foot perimeter of my present life and this is the most powerful tool in keeping my weight off.

CONNECTING GOALS

So how do we avoid trusting in maintenance? How do we move to the next level and keep our weight off? By making disciples of others and creating new goals. If you are nearing a desired weight by cutting back on calories and increasing exercise, perhaps your next goal could be to increase your cardiovascular strength. You could measure your improvement by checking your resting heart rate, blood pressure or simply in seeing how much resistance you can tolerate on a stationary bike or how quickly you finish a walk. Your goal would be separate from reaching a certain number on the scale but connected to the goal of weight loss simply because more intense exercise will help you keep the weight off. Increasing flexibility, strength in your torso, coordination and balance are additional areas of focus worth considering. They are separate, yet connected to the primary goal – increased, overall health. Clearly, the closer the connection to your original goal, the greater your chances for an enhancement to it.

Even after attaining all the physical goals you choose, you can continue increasing your health by considering other areas of health. Health does not just include physical well being. It has multiple planes including, emotional, spiritual, mental, social, and economic. Remember the first principle we covered,

Spirit, soul and body are connected and affect one another.

Since each area is connected and affected by the other in some form or fashion, they will all help us increase overall health.

The goal of adhering to a regular sleep routine could be a connecting goal for weight loss. Other examples of connecting goals for weight loss are increasing water intake, increasing fiber intake, cutting out fried foods, eating three servings of vegetables and two servings of fruit each day and monitoring the type of fat you consume (from saturated to unsaturated).

Be creative in your goal setting, stay connected to your original goal and reach for that next level of health. All the while, be looking for people with which to share your testimony, your success in weight loss and increased health. This is how you avoid the pitfall of maintenance.

Just keep one thing in mind as you continue with your goals,

If you focus on results you will never change, if you focus on the God who can change you, you will get results.

If I am keeping my goal of increasing intimacy with Jesus at the forefront of decreasing overeating, then weight loss is simply a byproduct of my larger goal. This goal for intimacy will then naturally lead to other smaller goals such as increasing time with my family, tithing, balancing work and rest. All of these, in turn, work together for the greater, more powerful goal.

> *"... being confident of this very thing, that He who has begun a good work in you will complete it until the day of Jesus Christ."*[4]

---

[1] 1 Corinthians 9:24-27, Philippians 2:12, Ephesians 4:11-16, Hebrews 5:12-6:1.

[2] Philippians 3:12–14.

[3] Matthew 28:19.

[4] Philippians 1:6.

· Chapter 22 ·

Expect the Unexpected

There is one last area that I must speak to before closing this book. It is important to warn you of a phenomenon I wasn't quite prepared for in my process of healing. After five years of work with God on my obsession with food, I have come to realize that food was a constant companion and I have slowly said 'good-bye' to her. She was a deceptive, untrustworthy attendant, but she was a companion that I leaned on for over twenty years. She brought me comfort, though fleeting. She brought me fantasy, though empty and bitter in the end. Regardless, she was familiar and the goodbye has been surprisingly hard.

I have always dreamed of this goodbye. But it is different from what I had imagined. I see myself now in a funeral parlor, decked in color and strength and the coffin at the front of the room is empty. It does not contain my favorite foods or my days of fasting and dieting. It is empty; for that is what my obsession consisted of – emptiness, promises never kept. This coffin is void of all that is good, all that is God.

In its place is reality. In its place are the facts that my life is riddled with fears and insecurities, failure I have ignored and relationships that failed. Without my old companion, I have had to face my reality. Thanks be to God, I do not face reality alone.

I cry more instead of less. I admit "I don't know" when before I played pretend. I hurt deeper and pray louder. I see things about my world that break my heart. My old companion kept me isolated and numb to a whole lot of truth. Now I am bare to it all. I used to think that I had a problem with food. Now I see that I had a problem with life on earth without God. Perhaps this season will end one day. Maybe it will continue. It doesn't matter to me.

If God took me back to the start of this process and gave me the chance to choose healing or numbness, I would choose the healing – that I now know. But I must give warning. You do not want to walk this path of healing without Jesus. As His holiness exposes your depravity, His mercy keeps you sane. In this place, you will gain a better glimpse of what it meant when He walked to Calvary. His love conquers all. I am a living testimony.

There is another side to this healing that I must also warn you about. It too came unexpectedly. Three years into my healing, a series of events took place that served as rewards only God could orchestrate. I fell in love with a wonderful, godly man at the age of 38, I married, became a step mom of two great young men and had my first baby.

Just as God's love is new every morning, I have come to see, every day, that I am a powerhouse for His kingdom. I am a spiritual dynamo. I have only begun to uncover the destiny God has in store for me and if I continue on this path of healing and new life, I will greatly affect my world.

At first blush these changes look inviting, but they can bring discomfort. For again, I am more familiar with the limits my obsession with food placed upon my life than I am with the freedom I have in Christ Jesus. Yet I continue in faith. I have laid down my drama and picked up His supernatural agenda. I see more visions and dream more dreams, I share more honestly and courageously with my friends, I am quicker to hug a child, to protect an animal from harm, and to speak out against injustice and empty religion.

Sometimes, when all of this change seems to be too much for me to stand, I go back to my old friend, food. I may overeat on chocolate or skip a couple meals in effort to lose weight. Thankfully, as a client recently realized, "At least I don't eat the whole bag!" This is progress.

Thank you for sharing in my progress. Thank you for reading about the hope of God in my life. I pray that you will love Him and depend on Him, finding Him in your full-length mirror.

Notes